"*The Relaxation and Stress Reduction Workbook* is both classic and contemporary. It has not only stood the test of time but also has kept up with changing times by including new research and evidence-based best practices."

—**Patrick Fanning,** coauthor of *The Daily Relaxer* and *Mind and Emotions*

"After seven editions, this workbook continues to be one of my favorite stress management resources. I still refer to my copy of the original version published in 1980. I love everything about this new edition, from the extensive references and strong theoretical framework to the practical, easy-to-use (and teach) self-help techniques. A must for anyone interested in stress management."

—**Richard Blonna, EdD**, retired professor emeritus from William Paterson
  University of New Jersey, and author of *Stress Less, Live More* and *Coping with
  Stress in a Changing World*

"*The Relaxation and Stress Reduction Workbook* is a classic. Its track record speaks for itself, now in its seventh edition and over one million copies sold. This is the 'go-to' workbook for stress reduction, offering a comprehensive array of strategies and down-to-earth practices to live better with stress and anxiety."

—**Bob Stahl, PhD**, coauthor of *A Mindfulness-Based Stress Reduction Workbook*,
  Living With Your Heart Wide Open, *Calming the Rush of Panic*, *A Mindfulness-Based
  Stress Reduction Workbook for Anxiety*, and *MBSR Every Day*

"*The Relaxation and Stress Reduction Workbook* is a classic that has helped millions of people to manage their stress and live happier, more relaxed lives. This latest edition contains updates that incorporate the latest research-based approaches and provide new tools and exercises to help you learn skills such as self-compassion, overcoming avoidance, and defusing negative thoughts to take away their power. Whether you are dealing with a difficult life transition; chronic work, health, or relationship stress; or daily hassles like traffic and paperwork that wear you down, this book will help you cope in healthy, positive ways."

—**Melanie Greenberg, PhD**, clinical psychologist and author of *The Stress-Proof Brain*

"This wonderful workbook will help individuals reduce their stress, as well as serve as a powerful tool for therapists. The exercises are beautifully laid out. The information is easy to follow, while having depth to the material that will make a difference in someone's life. Davis, Eshelman, and McKay provide an invaluable resource. I feel incredibly confident recommending this book to anyone wanting to decrease stress and improve psychological well-being."

—**Jonathan Barkin, PsyD**, partner, San Francisco Bay Area Center for Cognitive Therapy; assistant clinical professor at the University of California, Berkeley; and coauthor of *The Relaxation and Stress Reduction Workbook for Teens*

"I am so impressed with the thoroughness of the seventh edition of *The Relaxation and Stress Reduction Workbook*. It is a great resource for individuals and practitioners alike."

—**Michele Haney, PhD**, Red Rocks Community College, Denver, Colorado; coauthor of *Stress Owners' Manual*

The Relaxation & Stress Reduction WORKBOOK

SEVENTH EDITION

Martha Davis, PhD

Elizabeth Robbins Eshelman, MSW

Matthew McKay, PhD

New Harbinger Publications, Inc.

Publisher's Note

NEW HARBINGER PUBLICATIONS is a registered trademark of New Harbinger Publications, Inc.

Distributed in Canada by Raincoast Books

Copyright © 2019 by Martha Davis, Elizabeth Robbins Eshelman, and Matthew McKay
       New Harbinger Publications, Inc.
       5674 Shattuck Avenue
       Oakland, CA 94609
       www.newharbinger.com

Cover design by Amy Shoup

Acquired by Tesilya Hanauer

Edited by Brady Kahn

Indexed by James Minkin

All Rights Reserved
        Library of Congress Cataloging-in-Publication Data on file

Printed in the United States of America

24   23   22

10   9   8   7   6

We would like to dedicate this book to our families.

Thank you, Bill and Amanda, Don, Judy, Rebekah and Jordan.

Contents

Preface to the Seventh Edition

Today, we are inundated with all kinds of information, including a lot of information about stress and stress management. What is unique about this book is that it immediately zeros in on what is relevant to you, that is, the specific stressors in your life and how you react to them. Once you've identified the sources of your stress, your most disturbing symptoms, and how you typically cope with them, you are directed to the techniques that will help you in your particular situation. In short, you don't have to waste your time reading material that isn't relevant to your specific needs; instead, you can focus on simple step-by-step instructions that will teach you how to feel better now.

This workbook is based on more than thirty-five years of clinical experience working with clients who came to us with symptoms of tension and stress like insomnia, worry, high blood pressure, headaches, indigestion, chronic pain, depression, and road rage. When they seek help, many of these people report they are experiencing some kind of a transition, such as a loss, a promotion, or a move. This isn't surprising, since stress can be defined as any change to which you must adapt.

Most clients describe feeling worn down by everyday hassles such as dealing with inconsiderate or rude people, commuting long distances, caretaking children and elderly relatives, and managing tons of paperwork. One client referred to this wearing-down process as a "death by a thousand cuts." Indeed, unmanaged stress can have an accumulative effect that may lead to major psychological and physical illnesses. Clients also tell us about some of their less successful stress-management strategies: working harder and faster; numbing their pain and soothing themselves with drugs, alcohol, and food; worrying about their problems; procrastinating; and taking their frustrations out on others.

To date, over a million people have purchased this book to learn how to relax their bodies, calm their minds, turn around their self-defeating behavior, and take control of their hectic lives. Every so often we update this workbook, adding new strategies that the latest research and our clinical experience have shown to be effective. We eliminate techniques we've learned are not especially helpful, and we simplify and shorten some techniques, to save you time. This allows us to keep this workbook as an up-to-date, relevant resource for professionals, a solid source of information for individuals who want to learn to manage their stress on their own, and a popular textbook in classes and workshops on stress management and relaxation.

Recent research supports the commonsense notion that it is better to face your troubles than to run away from them. Although escaping painful feelings like anxiety, depression, and anger may make you feel better in the short run, in the long run, avoidance prevents you from having positive corrective experiences associated with facing these painful feelings. For example, dropping a speech class because you are worried about blowing a talk in front of a group of strangers may alleviate your anxiety immediately, but you don't get the experience of surviving giving the talk and the confidence that comes from learning that you can do it, albeit imperfectly. Instead, you continue to live in fear of public speaking, and the next time you are faced with giving a talk in front of a group, you are still terrified.

With this in mind, we've added some techniques to strengthen your ability to tolerate distressing feelings as well as build up your self-confidence so you can accomplish your goals more effectively. We've updated the "Body Awareness" chapter with new techniques and changed its name to "Body Scan." We've replaced the chapter "Focusing" with a chapter on self-compassion, which combines unconditional self-respect, self-care, and acceptance. We've revised the "Facing Worry and Anxiety" chapter (now called "Relieving Worry and Anxiety") by removing risk assessment and imagery exposure and adding the new coping strategy of defusion. We've replaced the chapter "Coping Skills Training for Fears" with a new chapter, "Facing Fear and Avoidance." This updated behavioral-based exposure program invites readers to disconfirm their fearful expectations with their actual experience during exposure exercises. We've updated the "Nutrition and Stress" and the "Exercise" chapters to keep pace with current guidelines.

Whether you want to make just a few changes in your lifestyle or you need a major life overhaul, this workbook shows you how to get started and stick with a program that is tailored for you. Based on the feedback we've received from our clients and readers who've used these techniques, your efforts will be amply rewarded.

Acknowledgments

The authors wish to acknowledge the following contributors to the seventh edition of this book. Their expertise, experience, and collaboration have made this a more valuable edition.

Caryl Fairfull, RD, is a registered dietitian and has held leadership positions in the American Academy of Nutrition and Dietetics. She is a graduate of the University of California at Santa Barbara in Nutrition and Dietetics and completed her dietetic internship at the Bronx VA Hospital in New York. She also holds a Master of Business Administration from the University of Santa Clara. Ms. Fairfull managed the Department of Nutrition Services for Kaiser Permanente's Santa Clara Medical Center. There she developed nutrition care guidelines and provided individual and group nutrition counseling. She later provided clinical services at Sierra Nevada Memorial Hospital in Grass Valley, California, where she is currently retired. Ms. Fairfull wrote chapter 19, "Nutrition and Stress."

Cheryl D. Pierson, PT, MS. Ms. Pierson's forty years in the health care field include experience as a clinician, manager, teacher, researcher, and consultant. She is a core faculty member of the Kaiser Permanente Neurologic Physical Therapy Residency. Community service is the passion that sustains her continued work as a mentor and educator. Her studies at the School of Lost Borders have reinforced her belief in the healing quality of community service. Ms. Pierson volunteers with SonRise Equestrian Foundation serving children with special needs. She is training to become a facilitator with the Connected Horse Project, which supports people affected by dementia and their caregivers. Ms. Pierson wrote chapter 20, "Exercise."

Pat Fanning is a professional writer in the mental health field. He has authored or coauthored eight self-help books, including *Self-Esteem, Thoughts and Feelings,* and *Mind and Emotions.* Mr. Fanning wrote chapter 11, "Self-Compassion."

The authors would like to thank Albert Ellis, PhD, for volunteering to review and give feedback on the "Refuting Irrational Ideas" chapter. Dr. Ellis developed rational emotive behavior therapy, upon which this chapter is based.

How to Get the Most Out of This Workbook

This workbook teaches you clinically proven stress-management and relaxation techniques. Each technique is presented with concise background information followed by step-by-step exercises. As you practice these techniques, you will gain new insight into your personal stress response and learn how to reestablish balance and a sense of well-being in your life.

Use this workbook as a guide. Read chapters 1 and 2 first. They are the foundation upon which all of the other chapters are built. Then you will know enough about stress and your personal reactions to stress to decide which chapters will be most helpful for you to read next.

Chapters 3 through 10 teach techniques for relaxation. Chapters 11 through 15 will help you with your stressful thoughts and feelings. Chapter 16 assists you in managing your time more effectively so that you can free up time to relax and do more of what is most important to you. From chapter 17 you can learn to communicate more assertively, and chapter 18 gives you many options to deal with environmental and interpersonal stress at work. Chapters 19 and 20 teach the basics of nutrition and exercise. Chapter 21 gives you some suggestions on how to increase motivation, deal with problems that come up along the way, and stick to your plan. There are also a host of materials available for download at the website for this book: http://www.newharbinger.com/43348. (See the very back of this book for more details.)

Stress and tension are present in your life every day. Stress management and relaxation can be effective only if you make them a daily part of your lifestyle. As you are learning the skills in this book that are pertinent to you, practice them repeatedly to ensure that you will be able to carry them out anytime you need to, without having to refer to written materials. Regular conscious practice can lead to habits of regular relaxation and stress reduction at an unconscious level.

Here are some suggestions that will help you relax on a regular basis:

- Make an agreement with yourself to set aside a specific time each day dedicated to relaxation. If finding the time to do the exercises in this book is an issue, read chapter 16 on time management.

- The length of time required each day to practice the relaxation techniques in this workbook varies. Start small. Doing a relaxation exercise for five minutes on a regular basis is better than doing it only once for an hour. Aim for twenty to thirty minutes of relaxation time once or twice a day. Note that some people prefer to take more frequent, shorter relaxation breaks.

- You decide when is the best time to relax based on your schedule by answering these two questions: When do you need to relax most? When can you realistically break away from external demands to take some time for yourself? Here are some examples of what clients in our stress-management and relaxation classes have found most helpful and doable:

  - Beginning the day with a relaxation exercise makes people more focused and proactive in dealing with the stressful demands of their day.

  - Taking a relaxation break during the day can reverse growing tension that would otherwise culminate in painful symptoms such as a headache or indigestion.

  - Relaxing before leaving work or upon arriving at home allows you to let go of and decompress from the tensions of your busy day and to become calm and revitalized enough to enjoy personal time at home.

  - Using a relaxation exercise to go to sleep quickly and then sleep soundly can result in waking up refreshed.

- Choose a quiet place where you will not be interrupted to learn the techniques. Once mastered, many of the relaxation techniques presented in this workbook can be done in stressful situations.

- Since this is a new activity for you, it is a good idea to let people around you know what you are doing. Ask them to help out by leaving you alone without distracting you. Family members, fellow office workers, and friends are usually very supportive of these exercises once they understand what you are doing and why.

- It's best not to practice a relaxation exercise right after eating a big meal or when very tired, unless your purpose is to fall asleep.

- You will enjoy your experience more if you choose a comfortable position in a location that has a comfortable temperature, wear loose clothing, and remove your contacts or glasses.

See your health care provider before beginning the work in this book if any of the following circumstances are relevant to you:

- You are over thirty or your reaction to stress involves physical symptoms, such as frequent headaches, stomach problems, or high blood pressure; your doctor should perform a physical examination to rule out possible physical problems that may need medical attention.

- After starting your stress-management program, you experience any prolonged negative physical effects.

- You have been taking medication that you may no longer need once your stress-related symptoms go away with regular practice of these exercises.

Your health care provider can be a supportive partner in your efforts to live a healthier life.

CHAPTER 1

How You React to Stress

Stress is an everyday fact of life. You can't avoid it. Stress results from any change you must adapt to, ranging from the negative extreme of actual physical danger to the exhilaration of falling in love or achieving some long-desired success. In between, day-to-day living confronts even the most well-managed life with a continuous stream of potentially stressful experiences. Not all stress is bad. In fact, stress is not only desirable but also essential to life. Whether the stress you experience is the result of major life changes or the cumulative effect of minor everyday hassles, it is how you respond to these events that determines the impact that stress will have on your life.

Sources of Stress

You experience stress from four basic sources:

1. Your environment bombards you with demands to adjust. You must endure weather, pollens, noise, traffic, and air pollution.

2. You also must cope with social stressors, such as demands for your time and attention, job interviews, deadlines and competing priorities, work presentations, interpersonal conflicts, financial problems, and the loss of loved ones. You have to interact with a barrage of email, messages, social media, and the Internet on a daily basis.

3. A third source of stress is physiological. The rapid growth of adolescence; the changes menopause causes in women; lack of exercise, poor nutrition, and inadequate sleep; and illness, injuries, and aging all tax the body. Your physiological reaction to environmental and social threats and changes also can result in stressful symptoms, such as muscle tension, headaches, stomach upset, anxiety, and depression.

4. The fourth source of stress is your thoughts. Your brain interprets complex changes in your environment and body and determines when to turn on the stress response. How you interpret and label your present experience and what you predict for your future can serve either to relax or to stress you. For example, interpreting a sour look from your boss to mean that

you are doing an inadequate job is likely to be anxiety provoking. Interpreting the same look as tiredness or preoccupation with personal problems will not be as worrisome.

Stress researchers Lazarus and Folkman (1984) have argued that stress begins with your appraisal of a situation. You first ask how dangerous or difficult the situation is and what resources you have to help you cope with it. Anxious, stressed people often decide that (1) an event is dangerous, difficult, or painful and (2) they don't have the resources to cope.

Fight-or-Flight Response

Walter B. Cannon, a physiologist, laid the groundwork for the modern meaning of stress at Harvard in the beginning of the twentieth century. He was the first to describe the *fight-or-flight response* as a series of biochemical changes that prepare you to deal with threat or danger. Primitive people needed quick bursts of energy to fight or flee predators like saber-toothed tigers. You can thank this response for enabling your ancestors to survive long enough to pass on their genetic heritage to you. Think of occasions in your life when the fight-or-flight response served you well, such as when you had to respond quickly to a car that cut in front of you on the freeway or when you had to deal with an overly aggressive panhandler. These days, however, when social custom prevents you from either fighting or running away, this "emergency" or *stress response* is rarely useful.

Hans Selye (1978), the first major researcher on stress, was able to trace what happens in the body during the fight-or-flight response. He found that any stressor, imagined or real, can cause the brain to send an alarm to the hypothalamus (the main switch for the stress response, located in the midbrain). The hypothalamus stimulates the sympathetic nervous system as well as the adrenal gland and pituitary gland, which are responsible for secreting the main stress hormones, adrenaline, norepinephrine, and cortisol. This sets in motion a series of changes in the body. These changes include the following: heart rate, breathing rate, muscle tension, metabolism, and blood pressure all increase. The hands and feet become cold as blood is directed away from the extremities and digestive system into the larger muscles that can help to fight or run. Sugar is released into the bloodstream to fuel a burst of energy. Some people experience butterflies in their stomachs. The diaphragm and anus lock. The pupils dilate to sharpen vision, and hearing becomes more acute. Physical processes not essential to the fight-or-flight response are put on hold. For instance, digestion, reproduction, growth, tissue repair, and the response of the immune and inflammatory systems are inhibited.

Fortunately, the same mechanism that turns the stress response on can turn it off. This is called the *relaxation response.* As soon as you decide that a situation is no longer dangerous, your brain stops sending emergency signals to your brain stem, which in turn ceases to send panic messages to your nervous system. Three minutes after you shut off the danger signals, the fight-or-flight response burns out. Your metabolism, heart rate, breathing rate, muscle tension, and blood pressure all return to their normal levels. Herbert Benson (2000) suggests that you can use your mind to change your physiology for the better, improving your health and perhaps reducing your need for medication in the process. He coined the term "the relaxation response" to refer to this natural restorative response.

Chronic Stress and Disease

Chronic or persistent stress can occur when life stressors are unrelenting, as they are, for example, during a major reorganization or downsizing at work, while undergoing a messy divorce, or when coping with chronic pain or disease or a life-threatening illness. Chronic stress also takes place when small stressors accumulate and you are unable to recuperate from any one of them. As long as the mind perceives a threat, the body remains aroused. If your stress response remains turned on, your chances of getting a stress-related disease may be increasing.

Researchers have been looking at the relationship between stress and disease for over a hundred years. They have observed that people suffering from stress-related disorders tend to show hyperactivity in a particular preferred system, or stress-prone system, such as the skeletomuscular, cardiovascular, or gastrointestinal system. For example, chronic stress can result in muscle tension and fatigue for some people. For others, it can contribute to stress hypertension (high blood pressure), migraine headaches, ulcers, or chronic diarrhea.

Almost every system in the body can be damaged by stress. When an increase in corticoids suppresses the reproduction system, this can cause *amenorrhea* (cessation of menstruation) and failure to ovulate in women, impotency in men, and loss of libido in both. Stress-triggered changes in the lungs increase the symptoms of asthma, bronchitis, and other respiratory conditions. Loss of insulin during the stress response may be a factor in the onset of adult diabetes. Stress suspends tissue repair and remodeling, which, in turn, causes decalcification of the bones, osteoporosis, and susceptibility to fractures. The inhibition of immune and inflammatory systems makes you more susceptible to colds and flu and can exacerbate some specific diseases such as cancer and AIDS. In addition, a prolonged stress response can worsen conditions such as arthritis, chronic pain, and diabetes. There are also some indications that the continued release and depletion of norepinephrine during a state of chronic stress can contribute to depression and anxiety.

The relationship between chronic stress, disease, and aging is another area of research. Experts in aging are looking at the changing patterns of disease and the emergence of degenerative disorders. Over just a few generations, the threat of infectious diseases such as typhoid, pneumonia, and polio has been replaced with such modern plagues as cardiovascular disease, cancer, arthritis, respiratory disorders like asthma and emphysema, and a pervasive incidence of depression. As you age normally, you expect a natural slowing down of your body's functioning. But many of these mid- to late-life disorders are stress-sensitive diseases. Currently, researchers and clinicians are asking how stress accelerates the aging process and what can be done to counteract this process.

Impact of Recent Experience

Thomas Holmes, MD, and his research associates at the University of Washington found that people are more likely to develop illnesses or clinical symptoms after experiencing a period of time when they've had to adapt to many life-changing events.

Dr. Holmes and his associates developed the Schedule of Recent Experience, which allows you to quantify how many changes you've experienced in the past year and consider how these stressful events may have increased your vulnerability to illness. The main purpose of this scale, however, is to increase your awareness of stressful events and their potential impact on your health so that you can take steps to reduce the level of stress in your life.

Schedule of Recent Experience

Instructions: Think about each possible life event listed below and decide how many times, if at all, each has happened to you within the last year. Write that number (from 0 to 4) in the Number of Times column. (Note that if an event happened more than four times, you would still give it a 4 in that column.)

Event	Number of Times (0–4)	x	Mean Value	=	Your Score
1. A lot more or a lot less trouble with the boss.		x	23	=	
2. A major change in sleeping habits (sleeping a lot more or a lot less or a change in time of day when you sleep).		x	16	=	
3. A major change in eating habits (eating a lot more or a lot less or very different meal hours or surroundings).		x	15	=	
4. A revision of personal habits (dress, manners, associations, and so on).		x	24	=	
5. A major change in your usual type or amount of recreation.		x	19	=	
6. A major change in your social activities (e.g., clubs, dancing, movies, visiting, and so on).		x	18	=	
7. A major change in religious activities (attending services a lot more or a lot less than usual).		x	19	=	

8. A major change in the number of family get-togethers (a lot more or a lot fewer than usual).		x	15	=
9. A major change in your financial state (a lot worse off or a lot better off).		x	38	=
10. Trouble with in-laws.		x	29	=
11. A major change in the number of arguments with your spouse (a lot more or a lot fewer than usual regarding child rearing, personal habits, and so on).		x	35	=
12. Sexual difficulties.		x	39	=
13. Major personal injury or illness.		x	53	=
14. Death of a close family member (other than spouse).		x	63	=
15. Death of spouse.		x	100	=
16. Death of a close friend.		x	37	=
17. Gaining a new family member (through birth, adoption, oldster moving in, and so on).		x	39	=
18. Major change in the health or behavior of a family.		x	44	=
19. Change in residence.		x	20	=
20. Detention in jail or other institution.		x	63	=
21. Minor violations of the law (traffic tickets, jaywalking, disturbing the peace, and so on).		x	11	=
22. Major business readjustment (merger, reorganization, bankruptcy, and so on).		x	39	=

23. Marriage.		x	50	=
24. Divorce.		x	73	=
25. Marital separation from spouse.		x	65	=
26. Outstanding personal achievement.		x	28	=
27. Son or daughter leaving home (marriage, attending college, and so on).		x	29	=
28. Retirement from work.		x	45	=
29. Major change in working hours or conditions.		x	20	=
30. Major change in responsibilities at work (promotion, demotion, lateral transfer).		x	29	=
31. Being fired from work.		x	47	=
32. Major change in living conditions (building a new home or remodeling, deterioration of home or neighborhood).		x	25	=
33. Spouse beginning or ceasing to work outside the home.		x	26	=
34. Taking out a mortgage or loan for a major purchase (purchasing a home or business and so on).		x	31	=
35. Taking out a loan for a lesser purchase (a car, TV, freezer, and so on).		x	17	=
36. Foreclosure on a mortgage or loan.		x	30	=
37. Vacation.		x	13	=

38. Changing to a new school.		x	20	=	
39. Changing to a different line of work.		x	36	=	
40. Beginning or ceasing formal schooling.		x	26	=	
41. Marital reconciliation with mate.		x	45	=	
42. Pregnancy.		x	40	=	
Your total score					

Scoring:

- Multiply the mean value by the number of times an event happened, and enter the result in the Your Score column for each event.

- Add up your scores to get your total score and enter it at the bottom of the schedule.

- For accurate scoring, remember that 4 is the highest number that can be used in the Number of Times column.

According to Dr. Holmes and his associates, the higher your total score, the greater your risk of developing stress-related symptoms or illnesses. Of those with a score of over 300 for the past year, almost 80 percent will get sick in the near future; of those with a score of 200 to 299, about 50 percent will get sick in the near future; and of those with a score of 150 to 199, only about 30 percent will get sick in the near future. A score of less than 150 indicates that you have a low chance of becoming ill. So, the higher your score, the harder you should work to stay well.

Because people vary in their perception of a given life event as well as in their ability to adapt to change, we recommend that you use this standardized test only as a rough predictor of your increased risk.

Stress can be cumulative. Events from two years ago may still be affecting you now. If you think that past events may be a factor for you, repeat this test for the events of the preceding year and compare your scores. Visit http://www.newharbinger.com/43348 to download this Schedule of Recent Experience.

Prevention

Here are some ways you can use the Schedule of Recent Experience to maintain your health and prevent illness. You can use it to:

1. Remind yourself of the amount of change that has happened to you by posting the Schedule of Recent Experience where you and your family can see it easily.

2. Think about the personal meaning of each change that's taken place for you and try to identify some of the feelings you experienced.

3. Think about ways that you can best adjust to each change.

4. Take your time when making decisions.

5. Try to anticipate life changes and plan for them well.

6. Pace yourself. Don't rush. It will get done.

7. Take time to appreciate your successes, and relax.

8. Be compassionate and patient with yourself. It is not uncommon for people to become overwhelmed by all the stresses in their lives. It takes a while to put into effect coping strategies to deal with stress.

9. Acknowledge what you can control and what you cannot control and, when possible, choose which changes you take on.

10. Try out the stress-management and relaxation techniques presented in this book and incorporate the ones that work best for you into your personalized stress-management program.

Symptom Relief

The major objective of this workbook is to help you achieve symptom relief using relaxation and stress reduction techniques. Complete the following checklist to determine exactly which symptoms you want to work on.

Symptoms Checklist

Use this checklist to record the symptoms that you want to work on now. After you've used this workbook to master the stress reduction techniques that work best for your symptoms, you can return to this checklist and use it to measure your symptom relief.

Instructions: Rate your stress-related symptoms below for the degree of discomfort that they cause you, using this 10-point scale:

Slight discomfort			Moderate discomfort				Extreme discomfort		
1	2	3	4	5	6	7	8	9	10

Symptom (Disregard those that you do not experience.)	Degree of discomfort (1–10) now	Degree of discomfort (1–10) after mastering relaxation and stress reduction techniques
Anxiety in specific situations		
Tests		
Deadlines		
Competing priorities		
Interviews		
Public Speaking		
Other		
Anxiety in personal relationships		
Spouse		
Parents		
Children		
Other		

Symptom (Disregard those that you do not experience.)	Degree of discomfort (1–10) now	Degree of discomfort (1–10) after mastering relaxation and stress reduction techniques
Worry		
Depression		
Anxiety		
Anger		
Irritability		
Resentment		
Phobias		
Fears		
Muscular tension		
High blood pressure		
Headaches		
Neck pain		
Backaches		
Indigestion		
Muscle spasms		
Insomnia		
Sleeping difficulties		
Work stress		
Other		

Important: Physical symptoms may have purely physiological causes. You should have a medical doctor eliminate the possibility of any such physical problems before you proceed on the assumption that your symptoms are completely stress-related.

Tactics for Coping with Stress

As a member of modern society, you have available to you a variety of methods to cope with the negative effects of stress. Doctors can treat your stress-related symptoms and diseases. Over-the-counter remedies can reduce your pain, help you sleep, keep you awake, enable you to relax, and counter your acid indigestion and nervous bowels. You can consume food, alcohol, and recreational drugs to help block feelings of discomfort. You may have diversions such as TV, movies, the Internet, hobbies, and sports. You can withdraw from the world into your home and avoid all but the most necessary contact with the stressful world around you.

Our culture rewards people who deal with their stress by working harder and faster to produce more in a shorter time. There are people who thrive in our rapid-paced culture who are referred to as *type A personalities*. The type A personality is a term that was coined in the 1970s to describe people who have a strong sense of time urgency, can't relax, are insecure about their status, are highly competitive, and are easily angered when they don't get their own way. The classic study of type A personality was the twelve-year longitudinal study of over 3,500 healthy middle-aged men reported by Friedman and Rosenman in 1974, which estimated that type A behavior doubled the risk of coronary heart disease. Although this popular concept has received a great deal of interest in health psychology, recent research (Williams 2001) has indicated that only the hostility component of type A personality is a significant health-risk factor.

An article presented in the *American Journal of Cardiology* (Denollet et al. 2006) discussed how certain personal traits can hurt heart health and proposed a new personality construct, referred to as type D or *distressed* personality. Type D behavior is characterized by the tendency to experience negative emotions (anger and hostility) and to inhibit these emotions while avoiding social contact with others. Both negativity and social withdrawal are associated with greater *cortisol* (a hormone that is closely related to cortisone in its physiological effects), increased reactivity to stress, and risk for coronary heart disease and other stress-related diseases. However, it is anyone's guess whether the type D label will have the staying power that the type A label has had.

In contrast to anxious, chronically stressed people, certain people are less vulnerable to stress, according to University of Chicago research psychologist Suzanne Kobasa and colleagues (1985). These stress-hardy individuals have a lower frequency of illness and work absenteeism. They view stressors as challenges and chances for new opportunities and personal growth rather than as threats. They feel in control of their life circumstances, and they perceive that they have the resources to make choices and influence events around them. They also have a sense of commitment to their homes, families, and work that makes it easier for them to be involved with other people and in other activities. According to Herbert Benson and Eileen Stuart, authors of *The Wellness Book* (1993), the incidence of illness is lowest in individuals who have these stress-hardy characteristics and who also have a good social support system, exercise regularly, and maintain a healthy diet.

In his popular book *Emotional Intelligence* (2005), Daniel Goleman refers to emotionally healthy people as individuals who consistently demonstrate self-awareness, self-discipline, and empathy. Goleman asserts through his book that emotional intelligence contributes to a person's ability to cope with stress.

In her book *The Tending Instinct* (2002), psychologist Shelley E. Taylor discusses how we are biologically programmed to care for one another. In her research, Taylor discovered that studies involving the fight-or-flight response involved only male subjects. She set out to see whether men and women deal with stress differently, and if so, how. She found that in times of stress, people (especially women) who are driven to turn to their social support group to give and receive support— instead of running or fighting—are much less likely to experience a prolonged stress response. Her theory is known as "tend and befriend." Taylor says, "Social ties are the cheapest medicine we have" (165).

Tactics for Coping with Stress Inventory

Before you embark on a program of change, it is important to consider how you currently manage your stress.

Instructions: Listed below are some common ways of coping with stressful events. Mark those that are characteristic of your behavior or that you use frequently.

_____   1. I ignore my own needs and just work harder and faster.

_____   2. I seek out friends for conversation and support.

_____   3. I eat more than usual.

_____   4. I engage in some type of physical exercise.

_____   5. I get irritable and take it out on those around me.

_____   6. I take a little time to relax, breathe, and unwind.

_____   7. I smoke a cigarette or drink a caffeinated beverage.

_____   8. I confront my source of stress and work to change it.

_____   9. I withdraw emotionally and just go through the motions of my day.

_____   10. I change my outlook on the problem and put it in a better perspective.

_____ 11. I sleep more than I really need to.

_____ 12. I take some time off and get away from my working life.

_____ 13. I go out shopping and buy something to make myself feel good.

_____ 14. I joke with my friends and use humor to take the edge off.

_____ 15. I drink more alcohol than usual.

_____ 16. I get involved in a hobby or interest that helps me unwind and enjoy myself.

_____ 17. I take medicine to help me relax or sleep better.

_____ 18. I maintain a healthy diet.

_____ 19. I just ignore the problem and hope it will go away.

_____ 20. I pray, meditate, or enhance my spiritual life.

_____ 21. I worry about the problem and am afraid to do something about it.

_____ 22. I try to focus on the things I can control and accept the things I can't.

Adapted from the *Coping Styles Questionnaire.* © 1999 by Jim Boyers, PhD, Kaiser-Permanente Medical Center and Health Styles, Santa Clara, CA.

Evaluate your results: The even-numbered items tend to be more constructive tactics and the odd-numbered items tend to be less constructive tactics for coping with stress. Congratulate yourself for the even-numbered items you checked. Think about whether you need to make some changes in your thinking or behavior if you checked any of the odd-numbered items. Consider experimenting with some even-numbered items you haven't tried before. This workbook will assist you in making these changes.

Knowing Your Goal

The goal of stress management is not merely stress reduction. After all, wouldn't life be boring without stress? As mentioned earlier, there is a tendency to think of stressful events or stressors only as negative (such as the injury or death of a loved one), but stressors are often positive. For instance, getting a new home or a promotion at work brings with it the stress of change of status and new responsibilities. The physical exertion of a good workout, the excitement of doing something challenging for the first time, or the pleasure of watching a beautiful sunset on the last day of your vacation are all examples of positive stress.

Distress or negative stress occurs when you perceive that the challenge facing you is dangerous, difficult, painful, or unfair, and you are concerned that you may lack the resources to cope with it. You can actually increase your ability to deal with distress by integrating into your everyday life positive activities such as solving challenging problems, practicing regular exercise workouts and relaxation techniques, staying in touch with enjoyable social contacts, following sensible dietary practices, and engaging in optimistic and rational thinking, humor, and play.

Performance and efficiency actually improve with increased stress until performance peaks as the stress level becomes too great. Stress management involves finding the right types and amounts of stress, given your individual personality, priorities, and life situation, so that you can maximize your performance and satisfaction. By using the tools presented in this workbook, you can learn how to cope more effectively with distress as well as how to add more positive stress or stimulating challenges, pleasure, and excitement to your life.

Symptom-Relief Effectiveness

Now that you've identified the major sources of your stress, your stress-related symptoms, and your current tactics for dealing with stress, it is time to choose one or two symptoms that bother you the most and select the techniques that you will use to relieve them. Defining and achieving a specific goal will give you a sense of accomplishment and motivate you to continue using the tools and ideas that give you the positive change you are seeking. Because everyone reacts differently to stress, we can't tell you which techniques will work best for you. However, the chart on the following pages will give you a general idea of what to try first and where to go from there.

Chapter headings for each stress reduction method are across the top, and typical stress-related symptoms are listed down the side. As you can see, more than one stress reduction technique can be effective for treating most symptoms. The most effective techniques for a particular symptom are marked with a boldface X, while a smaller and lighter x indicates other helpful techniques for the same symptom.

The techniques fall into roughly two categories: relaxation techniques that focus on relaxing the body and stress reduction techniques that condition the mind to handle stress effectively. Your mind, body, and emotions are interrelated. In seeking relief from stress, you will obtain the best results by using at least one technique from each of these two broad categories. For example, if your most painful stress symptom is general anxiety, you might practice progressive relaxation and breathing exercises to calm your body and work on the exercises from chapter 12 on refuting irrational ideas and chapter 13 on relieving worry and anxiety to reduce your mental and emotional stress. If your results on the Tactics for Coping with Stress Inventory indicate that you do not engage in regular physical exercise and your diet is not good, you will also want to refer to chapters 19 on nutrition and 20 on physical exercise to learn how improving these tactics can reduce your general anxiety.

Read chapter 2 before you move on to other chapters. Body awareness is the key to everything else in this workbook, and without it, you cannot use any of these techniques effectively.

Further Reading

Amundson, M. E., C. A. Hart, and T. A. Holmes. 1986. *Manual for the Schedule of Recent Experience (SRE)*. Seattle: University of Washington Press.

Benson, H. 1985. *Beyond the Relaxation Response*. New York: Penguin Publishers.

———. 2000. *The Relaxation Response*. Updated and expanded ed. New York: HarperCollins.

Benson, H., and E. Stuart. 1993. *The Wellness Book: The Comprehensive Guide to Maintaining Health and Treating Stress-Related Illness*. Reprint ed. New York: Simon & Schuster.

Denollet, J., S. S. Pederson, C. J. Vrints, and V. M. Conraads. 2006. "Usefulness of Type D Personality in Predicting Five-Year Cardiac Events Above and Beyond Concurrent Symptoms of Stress in Patients with Coronary Heart Disease." *American Journal of Cardiology* 97 (7): 970–73.

Friedman, M., and R. Rosenman. 1974. *Type A Personality and Your Heart*. New York: Knopf.

Goleman, D. 2005. *Emotional Intelligence*. 10th anniversary ed. New York: Bantam Books.

Kobasa, S., S. Maddi, M. Puccetti, and M. Zola. 1985. "Effectiveness of Hardiness, Exercise and Social Support as Resources Against Illness." *Journal of Psychosomatic Research* 29 (5): 525–33.

Lazarus, R. S., and S. Folkman. 1984. *Stress Appraisal and Coping*. New York: Springer Publishing.

Lorig, K., H. Holman, D. Sobel, D. Laurent, V. Gonzalez, and M. Menor. 2012. *Living a Healthy Life with Chronic Conditions*. 4th ed. Palo Alto, CA: Bull Publishing.

Martin, P. R. 1998. *The Healing Mind: The Vital Links between Brain and Behavior, Immunity and Disease*. New York: St. Martin's Press.

McBrooks, C., K. Koizumi, and J. O. Pinkston, eds. 1975. *The Life and Contributions of Walter Bradford Cannon 1871–1945*. Albany: State University of New York Press.

Ornstein, R., and D. Sobel. 1995. *Healthy Pleasures*. Cambridge, MA: Perseus Books.

———. 2010. *The Healing Brain*. Los Altos, CA: Malor Books.

Rabin, B. 1999. *Stress, Immune Function and Health: The Connection*. New York: Wiley-Liss.

Sapolsky, R. M. 2004. *Why Zebras Don't Get Ulcers: The Acclaimed Guide to Stress, Stress-Related Diseases, and Coping*. 3rd ed. New York: Henry Holt and Company.

Selye, H. 1978. *The Stress of Life*. New York: McGraw-Hill.

Sobel, D. S., and R. Ornstein. 1998. *Mind and Body Health Handbook*. 2nd ed. New York: Time-Life Books.

Taylor, S. 2002. *The Tending Instinct*. New York: Times Books.

Williams, R. B. 2001. "Hostility (and Other Psycho-Social Risk Factors): Effects on Health and the Potential for Successful Behavioral Approaches to Prevention and Treatment." In *Handbook of Health Psychology*, edited by A. Baum, T. A. Revenson, and J. E. Singer. Hillsdale, NJ: Lawrence Erlbaum Associates.

Symptom-Relief Effectiveness Chart

Symptoms	Techniques							
	Body Scan	Breathing	Progressive Relaxation	Meditation	Visualization	Applied Relaxation Training	Self-Hypnosis	Autogenics
Anxiety in specific situations (tests, deadlines, interviews, presentations)		X	X	x	x	X	x	
Anxiety in your relationships (spouse, children, boss)		X	x				x	
General anxiety and worry		X	X	X	x	X		x
Depression		X		X				
Hostility, anger, irritability, resentment		X	x	x		X		x
Phobias, fears		X	X		x	X		
Muscular tension	X	X	X		x	x	x	X
High blood pressure		x	X	X				X
Headaches, neck pain, backaches		x	X	X	X	X	X	x
Indigestion		x	X	x			X	X
Insomnia, sleeping difficulties		x	X			X	X	x
Work stress		X	X			X		
Chronic pain		X	x	X	X	x	X	X

Brief Combination Techniques	Self-Compassion	Refuting Irrational Ideas	Relieving Worry and Anxiety	Facing Fear and Avoidance	Anger Inoculation	Goal Setting and Time Management	Assertiveness Training	Work-Stress Management	Nutrition and Stress	Exercise
x		x	X	X		X	x			
x		x	X	x			X			
x	X	X	X	x		X	x		x	X
	X	X		x		x	X		x	X
	x	X			X	X	X		x	X
		x	X	X		x	x		x	x
x					x	x				X
x					x	x	x		X	X
							x		x	X
x						x	x		X	x
									x	X
		X			x	x	x	X		
		x				X	x		x	X

CHAPTER 2

Body Scan

In this chapter you will learn:

- How to recognize tension in your body

- How muscle tension and emotional responses are related

- Exercises to help you recognize and let go of tension in your body

Background

In recent years, technology has increased our access to people and information as well as sped up our pace of life. It's easy to get caught up in the distractions of our external lives and fail to notice the tension in our bodies until it becomes so intense that it is painful.

The ability to recognize how your body reacts to the stressors in your life can be a powerful skill. Most people are more aware of the weather, the time of day, or their bank balance than they are of the tension in their own bodies. In many cases, your body registers stress long before your conscious mind does. For example, your neck and shoulder muscles are likely to tense up over the course of a stressful day at work, and you may not notice how painfully tight they are until the end of the day. Muscle tension is your body's way of letting you know that you are stressed, and body awareness is the first step toward acknowledging and reducing that tension that can lead to painful symptoms.

You can use the exercises in this chapter to turn inward and pay attention to the sensations in your body in the present moment. You will observe how sensations of tension are related not only to your external stressors but also to your emotions, thoughts, and actions. With this knowledge you can begin to let go of this tension and make wiser choices to take care of yourself in the midst of your stressful day.

Differentiating between your external awareness and internal awareness so you can separate the world from your physical reaction to it is important. *External awareness* includes all stimulation to the five senses from the outside world. *Internal awareness* refers to any physical sensation, feeling, emotional discomfort, or comfort inside your body. Much of the tension in your body isn't felt, because most of your awareness is directed toward the outside world. Below, you will learn about exercises designed to locate and explore your body tension.

The importance of body states, their effect on consciousness, and their relationship to stress have been emphasized for many centuries by Eastern philosophies such as Zen, hatha yoga, and Sufism. During the last century, the work of Wilhelm Reich, originally a student of Freud, kindled Western psychiatry's interest in the body's interaction with emotional conditions. Two other therapies that concentrate on the body and its relationship to emotional stress are Fritz Perls's gestalt therapy and Alexander Lowen's bioenergetics therapy. Both of these therapies work closely with the mind-body relationship. Becoming aware of how your body responds to stress will give you some important information about your personal stress response that you can then use to develop a stress-management plan.

In 1979, Jon Kabat-Zinn, a molecular biologist, founded the mindfulness-based stress reduction (MBSR) program at the University of Massachusetts Medical School. MBSR uses a combination of mindfulness meditation, body awareness, and yoga to help people become more mindful and aware. Kabat-Zinn's research showed that MBSR resulted in significant improvement in the symptoms of patients with anxiety and/or chronic pain. A large body of research has accumulated demonstrating the benefits of mindfulness for people dealing with stress, anxiety, depression, pain, and illness.

Body Inventory

The following exercises promote body awareness and will help you identify areas of tension in your body. The body has its own wisdom, and if you take the time to listen, you can better understand how external stressors and your thoughts, feelings, and tension interconnect.

Inner-Outer Shuttle

This exercise teaches you to discriminate between your internal and external experiences and assists with increasing your awareness in order to identify your stress response.

1. First focus your attention on the outside world. Start sentences with "I am aware of." (For example, *I am aware of the cars going by outside the window, papers moving, the coffee brewing, the breeze blowing, and the blue carpet.*)

2. After you've become aware of everything that is going on around you, shift to focusing your attention on your body and your physical sensations—your internal world. (For example, *I am aware of feeling warm, my stomach gurgling, tension in my neck, my nose tickling, and a cramp in my foot.*)

3. Shuttle back and forth between internal and external awareness. (For example, *I am aware of the chair pressing against my buttocks, the circle of yellow light from the lamp, my shoulders hunching up, the smell of bacon.*)

If you practice during your free moments throughout the day, the Inner-Outer Shuttle will allow you to separate and appreciate the real difference between your inner and outer worlds.

Body Scanning

This exercise will help increase your awareness of where you carry muscle tension in your body.

Close your eyes. Starting with your toes and moving up your body, ask yourself, *Where am I tense?* Whenever you discover a tense area, exaggerate it slightly to become even more aware of it. Notice the muscles in your body that are tense.

Letting Go of Your Body

This exercise increases your awareness of muscle tension and decreases the buildup of muscle tension.

Lie down on a rug or a firm bed and get comfortable. Pull your knees up until your feet rest flat on the floor (or bed) and close your eyes. Check yourself for comfort. (This may require shifting your body around.) Become aware of your breathing…feel the air move into your nose, mouth, and down your throat into your lungs. Focus on your body and let all of the parts come into your awareness spontaneously. What parts of your body come into awareness first? What parts are you less aware of? Become aware of which parts of your body you can feel easily and which parts of your body have little sensation. Do you notice any difference between the right and left side of your body?

Now become aware of any physical discomfort you are feeling. Become aware of this discomfort until you can describe it in detail. Focus and be aware of what happens to this discomfort. It may change…now scan your body for any residual tension or discomfort and let it go with each exhalation. Continue letting go for five to ten minutes, allowing your body to take over.

Stress-Awareness Diary

Some parts of the day are more stressful than others, and some stressful events are more likely to produce physical and emotional symptoms than others. Certain types of stressful events often produce characteristic symptoms. For this reason, keeping a record of stressful events, as well as symptoms that may have been a stress reaction, is useful. You can use the following blank form for your own diary; it can also be downloaded at http://www.newharbinger.com/43348.

Keep this diary for one week. Make a note of the time that a stressful event occurs and the time you notice a physical or emotional symptom that could be related to the stress.

The following Stress-Awareness Diary was recorded one Monday by Harry, a department store clerk.

Time	Stressful Event	Symptom
8:00 a.m.	Alarm doesn't go off, late for work, only had time for coffee	Slight headache, jittery
9:30 a.m.	Boss reprimands me for being late	
9:50 a.m.		Worry, depression, shallow breathing
11:00 a.m.	Customer is rude and insulting	
11:15 a.m.		Anger, tightness in stomach
12:20 p.m.	Only have ten minutes for lunch, eat some chips	
2:30 p.m.		Slight headache
3:00 p.m.	Presentation to senior manager	Nervous, sweating
5:00 p.m.	Heavy commute, late for dinner with family	
6:00 p.m.	Argument with son	Anger, pounding headache
6:35 p.m.	Wife defends son	Anger, tension in neck, back, and stomach
10:00 p.m.		Worry, not able to sleep

Stress-Awareness Diary

Date: _____ Day of the week: _____

Time	Stressful Event	Symptom

As you can see, the diary identifies how particular stressors result in predictable symptoms. An interpersonal confrontation after having just coffee for breakfast is followed by stomach tension. Rushing may cause *vasoconstriction* (tightening of the blood vessels), and eating virtually nothing all day is likely to cause low blood sugar for this man, who, not surprisingly, experiences anger and various physical symptoms when he arrives home to face more confrontation.

Things to consider are how long does your emotional response, worry, anxiety, or anger last? What does it do to the muscular tension in your body? You can use your Stress-Awareness Diary to discover and chart your stressful events and characteristic reactions.

Releasing Tension

The next exercise will help you open to each part of your body, notice any sensation that is present, and let go of tension in your body. You can do this exercise to release tension any time you feel stressed.

The Inner Exploration or Body Scan

Allow yourself to check in with your body and mind, and simply let any waves of thoughts, emotions, and physical sensations just be.

1. Begin by becoming aware of the rising and falling of your breath in your chest and belly. You can ride the waves of your breath and let it begin to anchor you to the present moment.

2. Bring your attention to the soles of your feet. Notice any sensation that is present there. Without judging or trying to make it different, simply be present with the sensation. After a few moments, imagine that your breath is flowing into the soles of your feet. As you breathe in and out, you might experience an opening or softening and a release of tension. Just simply observe.

3. Now bring your attention to the rest of your feet, up to your ankles. Become aware of any sensation in this part of your body. After a few moments, imagine that your breath, instead of stopping at the diaphragm, flows all the way down to your feet. Breathe into and out of your feet, simply noticing the sensations.

4. Proceed up your body in this manner with all the parts of your body—lower legs, knees, thighs, pelvis, hips and buttocks, lower back, upper back, chest and belly, upper shoulders, neck, head, and face. Take your time to really feel each body part and notice whatever sensations are present, without forcing them or trying to make them be different; then breathe into the body part and let go of it as you move on to your next body part.

5. Go back to your neck and shoulders or any part of your body that has pain, tension, or discomfort. Simply be with the sensations in a nonjudgmental way. As you breathe in, imagine your breath opening up any tight muscles or painful areas and creating more spaciousness. As you breathe out, imagine the tension or pain flowing out of that part of your body.

6. Return to the top of your head and scan your body one last time for any areas of tension or discomfort. Then imagine that you have a breath hole at the top of your head, much like the blowholes that whales or dolphins use to breathe. Breathe in from the top of your head, bringing your breath all the way down to the soles of your feet and then back up again through your whole body. Allow your breath to wash away any tension or uncomfortable sensations.

The entire body scan can take anywhere from a few minutes to thirty minutes. Ideally, try to allow for twenty to thirty minutes to complete a body scan each day.

To keep a convenient record of how you feel before and after doing any of the body-scanning exercises from this chapter, use the following Record of General Tension. This record is also available at http://www.newharbinger.com/43348.

Mary, a customer service representative, recorded the following.

Week of _____	Exercise	Before session	After session	Comments
Monday	Body Scanning	10	7	Hectic day; felt anxious
Tuesday	Inner-Outer Shuffle	9	6	Coworker was ill, increased workload; felt angry
Wednesday	Body Scanning	9	5	Workload still intense; felt worried
Thursday	Letting Go of Your Body	8	4	Coworker back; felt relief
Friday	Inner Exploration or Body Scan	9	4	Another hectic day; felt less overwhelmed
Saturday	Letting Go of Your Body	6	3	Busy day at home; felt less worry
Sunday	Inner Exploration or Body Scan	5	2	Good day; took long walk with a friend

Record of General Tension

Rate yourself on this 10-point scale before and after you do your body-scan relaxation exercises.

1	2	3	4	5
totally relaxed, no tension	very relaxed	moderately relaxed	fairly relaxed	slightly relaxed

6	7	8	9	10
slightly tense	fairly tense	moderately tense	very tense	extremely tense

Week of _____	Exercise	Before session	After session	Comments
Monday				
Tuesday				
Wednesday				
Thursday				
Friday				
Saturday				
Sunday				

As you use these body-scanning exercises, you will begin to recognize where your body stores muscular tension and what factors contribute to your muscular tension. With increased awareness, you can find ways to let go of the tension you discover on a daily basis. Along with the release of tension, you will experience increased energy and a sense of well-being. As you become more aware of subtle symptoms of body tension, you can take a brief relaxation break to avert more painful symptoms such as a headache or an angry outburst. This chapter is a building block for observing and reducing your stress response.

Further Reading

Benson, H. 2000. *The Relaxation Response.* Updated and expanded ed. New York: HarperCollins.

Borysenko, J. 2007. *Minding the Body, Mending the Mind.* Updated and revised ed. Cambridge, MA: DaCapo Press.

Goleman, D., and J. Gurin, eds. 1993. *Mind Body Medicine: How to Use Your Mind for Better Health.* Yonkers, NY: Consumer Reports Books.

Jaffe, D. 1986. *Healing from Within.* New York: Fireside.

Kabat-Zinn, Jon. 2013. *Full Catastrophe Living: Using the Wisdom of Your Body and Mind to Face Stress, Pain, and Illness.* Revised and updated ed. New York: Bantam Books.

Knaster, M. 1996. *Discovering the Body's Wisdom.* New York: Bantam Books.

Lorig, K., H. Holman, D. Sobel, D. Laurent, V. Gonzalez, and M. Menor. 2012. *Living a Healthy Life with Chronic Conditions.* 4th ed. Palo Alto, CA: Bull Publishing.

Lowen, A. 1994. *Bioenergetics.* New York: Viking-Penguin.

Perls, F., and F. S. Perls. 1981. *The Gestalt Approach and Eye Witness to Therapy.* New York: Bantam Books.

Scheller, M. D. 1993. *Growing Older, Feeling Better.* Palo Alto, CA: Bull Publishing.

Stahl, B., and E. Goldstein. 2010. A *Mindfulness-Based Stress Reduction Workbook.* Oakland, CA: New Harbinger Publications.

Stevens, J. O. 1971. *Awareness: Exploring, Experimenting, Experiencing.* Moab, UT: Real People Press.

CHAPTER 3

Breathing

In this chapter you will learn to:

■ Use breathing to increase your awareness of your inner experience

■ Use breathing to release tension and relax

■ Use breathing to reduce or eliminate symptoms of stress

Background

Breathing is the fundamental necessity of life that most people take for granted. With each breath of air, you obtain oxygen and release the waste product: carbon dioxide. Poor breathing habits diminish the flow of these gases to and from your body, making it harder for you to cope with stressful situations. Certain breathing patterns may actually contribute to anxiety, panic attacks, depression, muscle tension, headaches, and fatigue. As you learn to be aware of your breathing and practice slowing and normalizing your breaths, your mind will quiet and your body will relax. Breath awareness and good breathing habits will enhance your psychological and physical well-being whether you practice them alone or in combination with other relaxation techniques.

Let's examine a breath. When you inhale, air is drawn in through your nose, where it is warmed to body temperature, humidified, and partially cleansed. Your diaphragm, a sheetlike muscle separating the lungs and the abdomen, facilitates your breathing by contracting and relaxing as you breathe in and out.

Your lungs are like a tree with many branches (*bronchial tubes*) that carry air to elastic air sacs (*alveoli*). The alveoli have the balloonlike ability to expand when air is taken into the lungs and contract when air is let out. Small blood vessels (*capillaries*) surrounding the alveoli receive oxygen and transport it to your heart.

Your heart pumps oxygenated blood to all parts of your body. An exchange takes place in which blood cells receive oxygen and release carbon dioxide, a waste product that is carried back to your heart and lungs, and then exhaled. This efficient method of transporting and exchanging oxygen and carbon dioxide is vital to sustain life.

When you breathe, typically, you use one of two patterns: (1) chest or thoracic breathing, or (2) abdominal or diaphragmatic breathing.

Chest or *thoracic breathing* is a common malady of modern life that is often linked with lifestyle, stress, anxiety, or other forms of emotional distress. It is shallow and often irregular and rapid. When air is inhaled, the chest expands and the shoulders rise to take in the air. Chronic shallow chest breathing or frequent breath holding can be associated with chronic stress, tension, poor posture, tight clothing, purposely holding in the stomach and pushing out the chest, sedentary lifestyle, painful feelings, or long periods of focused attention in which people forget to breathe regularly.

Too little oxygen and a carbon dioxide buildup in the body associated with breath holding can contribute to feelings of fatigue and depression. Rapid, shallow chest breathing often associated with the stress response and anxiety can result in symptoms such as light-headedness, heart palpitations, weakness, numbness, tingling, agitation, and shortness of breath. Too much carbon dioxide is exhaled, and (due to an imbalance in oxygen to carbon dioxide levels in the blood) too little oxygen reaches the brain and other parts of the body. In acute or extreme cases, rapid chest breathing is easily recognized as hyperventilation, but milder and slower chest breathing can go unnoticed for years.

Abdominal or *diaphragmatic breathing* is the natural breathing of newborn babies and sleeping adults. Inhaled air is drawn deep into the lungs as the abdomen expands, making room for the diaphragm to contract downward. Air is exhaled as the abdomen and the diaphragm relax. Diaphragmatic breathing is deeper and slower than shallow chest breathing, as well as more rhythmic and relaxing. The respiratory system is able to do its job of producing energy from oxygen and removing waste products.

By increasing your awareness of your breathing patterns and shifting to more abdominal breathing, you can balance the oxygen and carbon dioxide blood levels in your body, normalize your heart rate, and reduce the muscle tension and anxiety present with stress-related symptoms or thoughts. Diaphragmatic breathing is the easiest way to elicit the relaxation response.

Symptom-Relief Effectiveness

Breathing exercises have been found to be effective in reducing generalized anxiety disorders, panic attacks and agoraphobia, depression, irritability, muscle tension, headaches, and fatigue. They are used in the treatment and prevention of breath holding, hyperventilation, shallow breathing, and cold hands and feet.

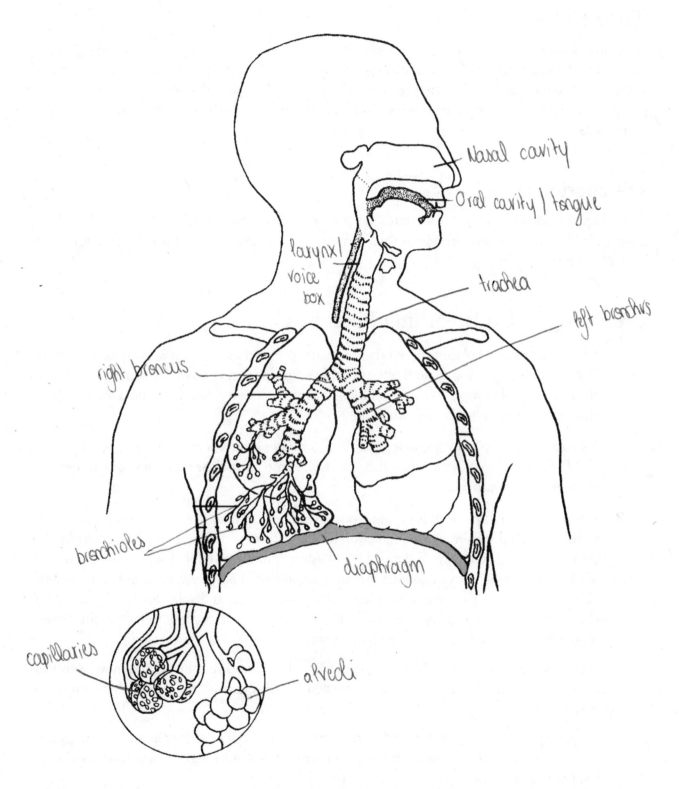

Nasal cavity

Oral cavity / tongue

larynx/ voice box

trachea

left bronchus

right bronchus

bronchioles

diaphragm

capillaries

alveoli

Adapted from W. Kapit and L. M. Elson (1977), *The Anatomy Coloring Book*, New York: Harper & Row.

Time to Master

A breathing exercise can be learned in a matter of minutes and some of its benefits experienced immediately. Regular practice of a breathing exercise can have profound effects in a matter of weeks, if not days. After you've tried the exercises presented in this chapter, develop a breathing program incorporating those exercises you find most helpful and follow your program daily for the best results.

Instructions

This chapter is divided into four sections: (1) preparing to do breathing exercises, (2) breathing basics, (3) breathing for tension release and increased awareness, and (4) breathing for symptom control or release.

Preparing to Do Breathing Exercises

1. Choose a time and place to learn these breathing exercises where you won't be disturbed. While you are learning to do them, try to do your daily practice in the same place and at the same time. However, a number of these exercises, once mastered, can be done anywhere you find yourself in a stressful situation.

2. It's best to breathe through your nose, unless otherwise instructed. If needed, clear your nasal passages before doing breathing exercises. If you can't clear them, it's okay to breathe through your mouth.

3. Think about what position is best for you. If your goal in practicing a breathing exercise is to be relaxed and maintain optimal awareness of your experience, do it from a seated position. If your goal is to relax and possibly fall asleep, practice it lying down. If you are seated while you do these exercises, remember to maintain good posture with your head comfortably balanced on your spine, your arms and legs uncrossed, and your feet firmly placed on the floor. Note that as a beginner, you will find it easier to learn how to breathe diaphragmatically lying down. Here are two lying down positions:

   If you have back problems, the *knees-raised pose* is best. Bend your knees and move your feet about eight inches apart, with your toes turned slightly outward. Make sure that your spine is straight.

   When you use the *dead-body pose*, lie on your back with your legs straight and slightly apart, your toes pointed comfortably outward, your arms at your sides and not touching your body, your palms are up, and your eyes are closed.

4. Whatever position you choose, take a moment to check in with yourself before beginning your breathing exercise. Scan throughout your whole body, releasing points of obvious tension, and shift your position, if necessary, to be more comfortable.

Breathing Basics

It is useful to observe how you are currently breathing before you learn how to use breathing as a relaxation skill.

How Do You Currently Breathe?

1. To answer the question "How do you currently breathe?" close your eyes. Put your right hand on your abdomen at the waistline, and put your left hand on your chest, in the center.

2. Without trying to change your breathing, simply notice how it feels as cool fresh air enters your nose, passes through the hairs in your nasal passage, reaches the back of your throat, and descends into your lungs.

3. Notice what happens as that breath of fresh air enters your lungs. What happens when you exhale? Observe your breath for a while without making any effort to make it different. Take your time.

4. Which hand rises the most when you inhale—the hand on your chest or the hand on your abdomen? If your abdomen expands and rises the most when you inhale, you are breathing diaphragmatically. If your abdomen doesn't move or if it moves less than your chest, you are shallow chest breathing.

Special Considerations

1. Once you become at ease with breathing diaphragmatically, check in with how you are breathing from time to time throughout your day. Are you breathing diaphragmatically? Shallowly? Are you holding your breath? Take a few diaphragmatic breaths. Concentrate on your abdomen moving up and down, the air moving in and out of your lungs, and the feeling of relaxation that deep breathing gives you. Then resume your normal activities.

2. If you have difficulty checking in with your breathing throughout the day, designate an external cue as a reminder to pay attention to your breath. An *external cue* is anything that you know you will notice at least several times a day: the steering wheel of your car, your office clock, or a sign posted on your door that says "Breathe."

3. When you've learned to relax using diaphragmatic breathing, you can use it to lower your tension level whenever you anticipate being in a stressful situation as well as during that situation and after that situation ends. Although it's not a panacea, most people report that diaphragmatic breathing helps them get through difficult situations more easily.

4. At first, diaphragmatic breathing may feel awkward, especially if you have been a shallow chest breather. As a beginner, it is useful to exaggerate the abdominal movement in this exercise in order to experience what it feels like. Once you have this movement down, you don't need to exaggerate it and you can place your hands at your sides. With practice, diaphragmatic breathing will feel more natural.

5. Diaphragmatic breathing is an integral part of most breathing exercises as well as part of most of the other relaxation techniques you will be learning in this workbook, so be sure that you've mastered it before moving on.

Diaphragmatic or Abdominal Breathing

1. Lie on your back and gently place one hand on your abdomen and one hand on your chest and follow your breathing. Notice how your abdomen rises with each inhalation and falls with each exhalation. Alternatively, put a book on your abdomen, place your hands at your sides, and follow your breathing.

2. If you experience difficulty breathing into your abdomen, try one of the following:

   a. Exhale forcefully to empty your lungs. This will create a vacuum that will pull a deep breath into your abdomen. If you find yourself drifting back to shallow chest breathing, you may need to repeat this.

   b. Press your hand down on your abdomen while you exhale and then let your abdomen push your hand back up as you inhale deeply.

   c. Imagine that your abdomen is a balloon and that as you inhale you are filling it with air.

   d. Lie on your stomach with your head resting on your folded hands. Inhale deeply into your abdomen so you can feel your abdomen pushing against the floor.

3. Is your chest moving in harmony with your abdomen or is it rigid? Although most of the action is in your abdomen when you breathe diaphragmatically, your chest does move a little. As you inhale, first your abdomen, then your middle chest, and then your upper chest will rise in one smooth movement. You might want to imagine filling a glass with water from the bottom to the top as you inhale.

4. Once you know what it feels like to breathe diaphragmatically, you can use this option to deepen and slow your breath even more. Smile slightly, inhale through your nose, and exhale through your mouth, as though you are breathing out through a straw. Take long, slow, deep breaths that raise and lower your abdomen. Focus on the sound and feeling of your breathing as you become more and more relaxed.

5. When thoughts, feelings, and sensations catch your attention, just notice them and return to your breathing.

6. Practice diaphragmatic breathing for about five or ten minutes at a time, once or twice a day. Gradually extend the time you do this to twenty minutes.

7. At the end of each diaphragmatic-breathing session, take a little time to notice (and enjoy) how you feel.

8. Optional: You may want to scan your body for tension at the beginning and end of each breathing practice session. Compare the level of tension you feel at the end of the exercise with the tension level you felt when you began. Use the Record of General Tension in chapter 2 to monitor your progress.

Breathing for Tension Release and Increased Awareness

Letting Go of Tension

1. Inhale diaphragmatically as you say to yourself, *breathe in*.

2. Hold your breath a moment before you exhale.

3. Exhale slowly and deeply as you say to yourself, *relax*.

4. Pause and wait for your next natural breath.

5. As you inhale slowly and then hold your breath for a moment, notice the parts of your body that tense up.

6. As you exhale, feel the tension naturally leaving your body. With each exhalation, you will feel more and more relaxed as you let go of more and more tension.

7. When thoughts, feelings, and sensations catch your attention, just notice them and return to your breathing.

8. Practice for five to twenty minutes at a time.

9. Once you've mastered this exercise, practice using it several times a day in neutral situations, that is, nonstressful situations. Finally, start using it in stressful situations to reduce your tension. Simply take several diaphragmatic breaths; say to yourself, *breathe in* and *relax*; and let go of the tension on the exhalation. Focus on the sensations of relaxation.

10. Remember that you may need to exhale before you can breathe in deeply.

Mindful Breathing

In the preceding exercises, you may have noticed that your mind tends to wander to bodily sensations, noises, daydreams, plans, worries, judgments, and so forth. This is natural, but it can hinder your ability to let go of the stresses in your life and thereby inhibit relaxation. Mindfully counting your breaths provides you with a way to observe your experience that will help you calm your mind as well as relax your body.

Being *mindful* means being aware of your experiences in the here and now as an objective and friendly observer without getting caught up in those experiences. An objective observer is like a scientist who steps back and looks at what is happening in an experiment without judgment or expectation, open to learning something new. A friendly observer is compassionate without being swept away by what is going on. Of course, this is easier said than done. Fortunately, the more you practice this mindfulness mind-set, the easier it becomes. In addition, each time you lose track of your point of focus (in this case, your breath and the counting of your breaths) and bring it back to your attention, you are strengthening your ability to attend.

Mindful Breath Counting

1. Practice this exercise sitting up to enhance mindfulness awareness. Later, if you like, you can use it in bed as a technique to help you fall asleep.

2. Use slow, deep diaphragmatic breathing.

3. Count each exhalation to yourself. When you reach the fourth exhalation, start over again at one. Here is how you do it: inhale…exhale (*one*)…inhale…exhale (*two*)… inhale…exhale (*three*)…inhale…exhale (*four*)…inhale…exhale (*one*)…and so forth.

4. As other thoughts enter your consciousness or as your mind goes blank, simply observe those thoughts or the blankness without judgment or expectation, and then return to counting your breaths.

5. If you lose track of your count, simply start over again at "one."

6. Optional: If you like, you can label each of your thoughts, feelings, and sensations as they arise. Say to yourself, *thought, feeling*, or *sensation*, and then return to counting your breaths. You can make up your own labels, but keep it simple. The purpose of labeling is to increase your objectivity and emotional distance from potentially charged material.

7. Continue counting your exhalations in sets of four for ten minutes. Gradually increase to twenty minutes.

Here is an example of a few moments of a beginner's experience with Mindful Breath Counting:

Inhale… *Remember to breathe into my belly…that's a thought…*exhale (*one*)…inhale…exhale (*two*)…inhale…exhale (*three*)… *My shoulders are really tight…sensations…thought…*inhale… exhale (*four*)…inhale… *Oh, it feels good to let go of that tension…sensation, feeling, thought…* exhale (*one*)…inhale…exhale (*two*)… *Did I lock the front door when I came home? Tension in my chest, holding my breath… Yes, relief…thoughts, sensations, feelings… I can't do this… thought, remember to breathe…now where was I?…more thoughts…* Inhale…exhale (*one*)….

To learn more about mindfulness, turn to chapter 5, "Meditation."

Note that when you practice any relaxation exercise and you find your mind has wandered, you can gently bring your attention back to your original point of focus. Adopting an objective and compassionate awareness of your experience in the here and now when you practice relaxation exercises can help you develop and strengthen these qualities in your everyday life. Once you have learned to return to your breath and your counting when you notice yourself being distracted, you may prefer to drop the counting and use your breath as the point of focus for your meditation.

Little Tension Releasers

During the day, there are many moments when you can benefit from a short time-out, such as when you catch yourself sighing or yawning. This is generally a sign that you are not getting enough oxygen. Since a sigh or a yawn actually does release a bit of tension, you can practice sighing or yawning at will as a way to relax. Make a conscious effort to sit or stand up straight when you do this.

Sighing

1. Sigh deeply, letting out a sound of deep relief as the air rushes out of your lungs.

2. Don't think about inhaling—just let the air come in naturally.

3. Repeat whenever you feel the need for it.

Yawning

1. Open your mouth wide.

2. Stretch your arms over your head.

3. Yawn (loudly if you can).

4. Repeat as needed.

Diaphragmatic Breathing

1. Step back mentally from what you are doing.

2. Notice how you feel.

3. Take three slow, relaxing, deep diaphragmatic breaths.

4. Notice how you feel.

5. Repeat as needed.

Note: Sometimes you don't have time to step back mentally and check in with yourself about how you're feeling. Nevertheless, you can still get a bit of tension release by breathing diaphragmatically a few times.

Breathing for Symptom Control or Release

The following exercise combines the relaxing benefits of diaphragmatic breathing with the curative value of positive *autosuggestion*, a thought or an image that influences your subjective experience.

Abdominal Breathing and Imagination

1. Place your hands gently on your solar plexus (the point where your ribs start to separate above your abdomen). Get comfortable and begin to relax as you breathe diaphragmatically for a few minutes.

2. Imagine that energy is rushing into your lungs with each incoming breath of air and being immediately stored in your solar plexus. Imagine that this energy is flowing out to all parts of your body with each exhalation. Make a mental picture of this energizing process.

3. Continue doing this exercise for at least five to ten minutes a day on a daily basis.

Alternatives to step 2:

Keep one hand on your solar plexus and move the other hand to a point on your body that hurts. As you inhale, imagine energy coming in and being stored. As you exhale, imagine the energy flowing to the spot that hurts and stimulating that spot. As you continue to inhale more energy, imagine this energy driving out the pain with each exhalation. Picture this process in your mind's eye.

Keep one hand on your solar plexus and move the other hand to a point on your body that has been injured or is infected. Imagine the energy coming in and being stored as you inhale. As you exhale, imagine that you are directing energy to the affected point and stimulating it, driving out the infection or healing it.

Most people will find this next relaxation exercise useful, but those suffering from tension or sinus headaches often find it particularly beneficial.

Alternate Nostril Breathing

Begin by doing five cycles, and then slowly raise the number to between ten and twenty-five cycles.

1. Sit in a comfortable position with good posture.

2. Rest the index and second finger of your right hand on your forehead.

3. Close your right nostril with your thumb.

4. Inhale slowly and soundlessly through your left nostril.

5. Close your left nostril with your ring finger and simultaneously open your right nostril by removing your thumb.

6. Exhale slowly and soundlessly and as thoroughly as possible through your right nostril.

7. Inhale through your right nostril.

8. Close your right nostril with your thumb and open your left nostril.

9. Exhale through your left nostril.

10. Inhale through your left nostril, beginning the next cycle.

The following Breath Training exercise, adapted from Masi (1993), has also been called *breathing retraining*. Individuals with panic disorder or agoraphobia find it particularly helpful. When most people feel panic, they have a tendency to gasp, take in a breath, and hold onto it. The resulting sensation of fullness and inability to get enough air in turn produces quick, shallow breathing or hyperventilation. Hyperventilation can trigger a panic attack. Breath training provides a crucial counting or pacing procedure to help counteract this process. Here are the steps to follow.

Breath Training

1. Exhale first. At the first sign of nervousness or panic, at the first *what if* thought that you might pass out, have a heart attack, or be unable to breathe, *always* exhale. It is important to exhale first so that your lungs open up and you'll feel as though there's plenty of room to take a good deep breath.

2. Inhale and exhale through your nose. Exhaling through your nose will slow down your breathing and prevent hyperventilation. If you can't breathe through your nose, inhale through your mouth and exhale slowly through your mouth by slightly pursing your lips and pretending that you are blowing out through a straw.

3. When you are first learning this technique, lie on your back with one hand on your abdomen and the other hand on your chest. Exhale first, and then breathe in through your nose, counting *one…two…three*. Pause for a second, and then breathe out through your mouth, counting *one…two…three…four*. Make sure that your exhalation is always longer than your inhalation. This will prevent you from taking short, gasping panic breaths.

4. After you feel comfortable doing step 3, you can slow your breathing even further. Breathe in and count, *one…two…three…four*; pause and breathe out, counting *one… two…three…four…five*. Keep practicing these slow, deep breaths, pushing the hand on your abdomen up but allowing very little movement for the hand on your chest. When your mind wanders, refocus on your breathing.

Alternative positions:

Lie on your stomach with your hands folded under your head. Continue to count *one…two… three* as you breathe in and *one…two…three…four* as you breathe out. As in step 4 above, breathe even more slowly by counting to four as you inhale and to five as you exhale.

Step 4 can also be done while you are standing, walking, or sitting. Pace your steps to match the same slow rate of your breathing.

When paced breathing feels comfortable and natural, you can replace counting with the words "in" as you inhale and "calm" as you exhale. Maintain the same pace, making each exhalation last slightly longer than each inhalation. Breathe in through your nose and breathe out through your mouth. Remember to always exhale first.

Final Thoughts

You will find it easier to relax your body, calm your mind, and cope with the stresses in your life when you practice a breathing relaxation exercise at least once or twice a day for twenty minutes. Make a plan right now to set aside time for this on a daily basis. In addition, remember to check in with your breathing from time to time throughout your day, especially when feeling stressed. If you catch yourself holding your breath or breathing shallowly or quickly, consciously take a few diaphragmatic breaths.

Further Reading

Airey, R. 2004. *Fifty Natural Ways to Better Breathing*. London: Anness Publishing.

Benson, H., and E. Stuart. 1993. *The Wellness Book: The Comprehensive Guide to Maintaining Health and Treating Stress-Related Illness*. Reprint ed. New York: Simon & Schuster.

Farhi, D. 1996. *The Breathing Book: Good Vitality Through Essential Breath Work*. New York: Owl Books.

Hendricks, G. 1995. *Conscious Breathing: Breathwork for Health, Stress Release, and Personal Mastery*. New York: Bantam Books.

Lewis, D. 2004. *Free Your Breath, Free Your Life: Conscious Breathing Can Relieve Stress, Increase Vitality, and Help You Live More Fully*. Boston: Shambhala Publications.

Recordings

Hendricks, G. 2005. *The Art of Breathing and Centering: Discover the Powerful Gifts of the Air You Breathe!* (Audio CD). New York: Audio Renaissance.

Lewis, D. 2005. *Natural Breathing* (3 Audio CDs). Louisville, CO: Sounds True.

Masi, N. 1993. *Breath of Life* (Audio CD). Plantation, FL: Resource Warehouse.

McKay, M., and P. Fanning. 2008. *Progressive Relaxation and Breathing* (Audio CD). Oakland, CA: New Harbinger Publications.

Weil, A. 1999. *Breathing: The Master Key to Self Healing* (Audio CD). Louisville, CO: Sounds True.

CHAPTER 4

Progressive Relaxation

In this chapter you will learn to:

- **Distinguish between tense and relaxed muscles**
- **Progressively relax all of the muscles of your body**
- **Relax quickly in stressful situations**

Background

You cannot have the feeling of warm well-being in your body and at the same time experience psychological stress. Progressive relaxation of your muscles reduces pulse rate, blood pressure, and the startle reflex, along with perspiration and respiration rates. Deep muscle relaxation, when successfully mastered, can be used as an antianxiety pill.

Edmund Jacobson, a Chicago physician, published the book *Progressive Relaxation* in 1929. In it he described his deep muscle relaxation technique, which he asserted required no imagination, willpower, or suggestion. His technique is based on the premise that the body responds to anxiety-provoking thoughts and events with muscle tension. This physiological tension, in turn, increases the subjective experience of anxiety. Deep muscle relaxation reduces physiological tension and is incompatible with anxiety: the habit of responding with one blocks the habit of responding with the other.

Jacobson's original progressive relaxation procedures might take many months or even years to learn, but Joseph Wolpe (1958) developed a short form for these procedures that included verbal suggestions to relax. This abbreviated form can be mastered in a matter of days or weeks. Wolpe made this streamlined version a part of his systematic desensitization protocol for the treatment of phobias. He found that once they relaxed, clients were more capable of tolerating and responding adaptively to situations they were afraid of.

Symptom-Relief Effectiveness

Excellent results have been found with progressive relaxation techniques for the treatment of muscular tension, anxiety, depression, fatigue, insomnia, neck and back pain, high blood pressure, mild phobias, and stuttering.

Time to Master

One to two weeks, employing two fifteen-minute sessions per day.

Instructions

Many people do not know which of their muscles are chronically tense. When you practice progressive relaxation, you focus on the sensations of tension in one particular muscle group at a time. Then, when you release that tension, you focus on the sensations of relaxation in that same muscle group. You move progressively through your whole body from one muscle group to the next, repeating this procedure. Using progressive relaxation techniques, you learn to identify particular muscle groups and to distinguish between the sensations of tension and deep relaxation.

Progressive relaxation can be practiced lying down or seated in a chair. Each muscle group is tensed from five to seven seconds and then released and relaxed for twenty to thirty seconds. These lengths of time are simply rules of thumb and don't have to be slavishly adhered to. This procedure is repeated at least once. If a particular muscle is difficult to relax, you can practice tensing and releasing it up to five times.

Once the procedure is familiar enough to be remembered, keep your eyes closed and focus your attention on just one muscle group at a time. Another option is to purchase a professional recording such as the one listed in the Recording section of this chapter.

The instructions for progressive relaxation are divided into two sections. The first part deals with the basic procedure, which you may wish to record and replay while practicing. This will familiarize you with the muscles in your body that are most commonly tense. If you do record these instructions, be sure to pause long enough for tensing and relaxing. The second section shortens the procedure by simultaneously tensing and relaxing many muscles at one time so that deep muscle relaxation can be achieved in a very brief time period.

The Three Basic Levels of Tensing

There are three basic levels of tensing that you can use when you practice progressive relaxation. With experience, you can decide which level of tensing is most pleasant and effective for your needs.

1. *Active tensing* involves tensing a particular muscle group as tightly as you can without hurting yourself, studying the sensations of tension, then releasing the tension and studying the sensations of relaxation in that same area. While you are tensing one part of your body, the rest of your body is relatively relaxed. Remember to breathe diaphragmatically (it's easy to forget to breathe this way, especially during the tensing phase). Active tensing is the level of progressive relaxation described in the Basic Procedure. By really exaggerating the tension, you are likely to feel where you carry chronic tension; the tense place may actually be sore. For people who have no injuries and who are not extremely tense, active tensing is recommended as the method of choice at least for the first time that you practice progressive relaxation. Some people prefer using this level every time they practice progressive relaxation, because tensing the muscles fatigues the muscle fibers and releasing the tension feels very relaxing and good. It's a little like setting down heavy bags you've been holding while standing in a long line.

2. *Threshold tensing* is the same as active tensing except that it involves tensing a particular muscle group only slightly (just enough so that you notice the tension; it's barely noticeable to the human eye). Threshold tensing should be used to avoid pain or injury for areas of your body that are injured or very tense. Many people prefer to use threshold tensing once they've become familiar with the basic muscle groups through active tensing because threshold tensing takes less effort and feels less invasive. Some people use threshold tensing from the beginning because of health issues or extreme tension.

3. *Passive tensing* is the same as active tensing except that during the tensing phase you simply notice any tension that is present in a particular muscle group. You can use the Basic Procedure described in this chapter and substitute the words "Notice the tension in your _____" whenever the instructions call for tensing a muscle. If you feel no tension in a particular muscle, do threshold tensing or simply notice the sensations that are there. You may prefer to use passive tensing on a regular basis once you are familiar with active and threshold tensing. You will find that a round of progressive relaxation using passive tension, following a round of either active or threshold tensing, can deepen your state of relaxation.

Verbal Suggestions

As you are releasing tension, you may also find it helpful to say to yourself one or more of the following expressions:

Let go of the tension.

Calm and rested.

Relax and smooth out the muscles.

Let the tension dissolve away.

Let go more and more.

Deeper and deeper.

Basic Procedure

Get into a comfortable position in a quiet room where you won't be disturbed. You may want to loosen your clothing and remove your shoes. Begin to relax as you take a few slow, deep breaths.... Now as you let the rest of your body relax, clench your fists and bend them back at the wrist...tighter and tighter...feel the tension in your fists and forearms.... Now relax.... Feel the looseness in your hands and forearms.... Notice the contrast with the tension.... (If you have time, repeat this, and all succeeding procedures, at least one more time.) *Now bend your elbows and tense your biceps.... Tense them as hard as you can and observe the feeling of tautness.... Let your hands drop down and relax.... Feel that difference.... Turn your attention to your head and wrinkle your forehead as tight as you can.... Feel the tension in your forehead and scalp. Now relax and smooth it out. Imagine your entire forehead and scalp becoming smooth and at rest.... Now frown and notice the strain spreading throughout your forehead.... Let go. Allow your brow to become smooth again.... Squeeze your eyes closed...tighter.... Relax your eyes. Let them remain closed gently and comfortably.... Now, open your mouth wide and feel the tension in your jaw.... Relax your jaw.... When your jaw is relaxed, your lips will be slightly parted. Notice the contrast between tension and relaxation.... Now press your tongue against the roof of your mouth. Experience the strain in the back of your mouth.... Relax.... Press your lips now and purse them into an "O."... Relax your lips.... Feel the relaxation in your forehead, scalp, eyes, jaw, tongue, and lips.... Let go more and more....*

Now roll your head slowly around on your neck, feeling the point of tension shifting as your head moves...and then slowly roll your head the other way. Relax, allowing your head to return to a comfortable upright position.... Now shrug your shoulders and bring your shoulders up toward your ears...hold it.... Drop your shoulders back down and feel the relaxation spreading through your neck, throat, and shoulders...pure relaxation, deeper and deeper....

Now breathe in and fill your lungs completely. Hold your breath. Experience the tension.... Now exhale and let your chest become loose.... Continue relaxing, letting your breath come freely and gently.... Notice the tension draining out of your muscles with each exhalation.... Next, tighten your stomach and hold. Feel the tension.... Relax.... Now place your hand on your stomach. Breathe deeply into your stomach, pushing your hand up. Hold...and relax. Feel the sensations of relaxation as the air rushes out.... Now arch your back, without straining. Keep the rest of your body as relaxed as possible. Focus on the tension in your lower back.... Now relax.... Let the tension dissolve away.

Tighten your buttocks and thighs.... Relax and feel the difference.... Now straighten and tense your legs and curl your toes downward. Experience the tension.... Relax.... Straighten and tense your legs and bend your toes toward your face. Relax.

Feel the comfortable warmth and heaviness of deep relaxation throughout your entire body as you continue to breathe slowly and deeply.... You can relax even more as you move up through your body, letting go of the last bit of tension in your body. Relax your feet...relax your ankles... relax your calves...relax your shins...relax your knees...relax your thighs...relax your buttocks.... Let the relaxation spread to your stomach...to your lower back...to your chest.... Let go more and more. Feel the relaxation deepening in your shoulders...in your arms...and in your hands.... Deeper and deeper. Notice the feeling of looseness and relaxation in your neck...your jaw...your face...and your scalp.... Continue to breathe slowly and deeply. Your entire body is comfortably loose and relaxed, calm and rested.

Shorthand Procedure

Once you have mastered the basic procedure, use the following procedure to relax your muscles quickly. In this procedure, whole muscle groups are simultaneously tensed and then relaxed. As before, repeat each procedure at least once, tensing each muscle group from five to seven seconds and then relaxing from fifteen to thirty seconds. Remember to notice the contrast between the sensations of tension and relaxation.

1. Curl both fists, tightening your biceps and forearms (Charles Atlas pose). Relax.

2. Roll your head around on your neck clockwise in a complete circle, then reverse. Relax.

3. Wrinkle up the muscles of your face like a walnut: forehead wrinkled, eyes squinted, mouth opened, and shoulders hunched. Relax.

4. Arch your shoulders back as you take a deep breath into your chest. Hold. Relax. Take a deep breath, pushing out your stomach. Hold. Relax.

5. Straighten your legs and point your toes back toward your face, tightening your shins. Hold. Relax. Straighten your legs and curl your toes, simultaneously tightening your calves, thighs, and buttocks. Relax.

Special Considerations

1. If you make a recording of the basic procedure to facilitate your relaxation program, remember to pause long enough for tensing and relaxing each muscle or muscle group before going on to the next muscle or muscle group.

2. As with all relaxation techniques, regular practice of progressive relaxation will enhance the speed and depth of your relaxation.

3. Be extra cautious when tensing your neck and back, because excessive tightening can result in muscle or spinal damage. Also, overtightening your toes or feet can result in muscle cramping.

4. People new to this technique sometimes make the error of relaxing tension gradually. This slow-motion release of tension may look relaxed, but it actually requires sustained tension. When you release the tension in a particular muscle, let it go instantly; let your muscles become suddenly limp.

5. Although initially you will learn progressive relaxation in a quiet place, eventually you will be able to use at least a shortened version of it anytime during the day when you notice you are tense.

Further Reading

Bernstein, D. A., T. D. Borkovec, and H. Hazlett-Stevens. 2000. *New Directions in Progressive Relaxation Training: A Guidebook for Helping Professionals*. New York: Praeger Publishing.

Bernstein, D. A., C. R. Carlson, and J. E. Schmidt. 2008. "Progressive Relaxation: Abbreviated Methods." In *Principles and Practice of Stress Management*, 3rd ed. Edited by P. M. Lehrer, R. L. Woolfold, and W. E. Sime. New York: Guilford Press.

Jacobson, E. 1974. *Progressive Relaxation*. Revised ed. Chicago: University of Chicago Press, Midway Reprint. Out of print.

McGuigan, F. J., and P. M. Lehrer. 2008. "Progressive Relaxation: Origins, Principles and Clinical Applications." In *Principles and Practice of Stress Management*, 3rd ed. Edited by P. M. Lehrer, R. L. Woolfold, and W. E. Sime. New York: Guilford Press.

Wolpe, J. 1958. *Psychotherapy by Reciprocal Inhibition*. Palo Alto, CA: Stanford University Press.

———. 1990. *The Practice of Behavior Therapy*. 4th ed. New York: Pergamon Press.

Recording

McKay, M., and P. Fanning. 2008. *Progressive Relaxation and Breathing* (Audio CD). Oakland, CA: New Harbinger Publications.

Meditation

Background

Meditation is the intentional practice of uncritically focusing your attention on one thing at a time. Exactly what that thing might be is relatively unimportant and varies from one tradition to the next. Often the meditator repeats, either aloud or silently, a syllable, word, or group of words. This is known as *mantra meditation*. Focusing on a fixed object such as a candle's flame or a flower can also anchor the attention. Many meditators find that a convenient and relaxing point of focus is the rising and falling of their own breath. But you can use anything as an object of meditation...the calendar on your desk, the tip of your nose, or even your Aunt Mary's maiden name.

It is important to understand that the heart of meditation lies not simply in focusing on one object to the exclusion of all other thought but rather in the attempt to achieve this type of focus. The nature of the mind is such that it does not want to stay concentrated. A myriad of thoughts will appear and seemingly interfere with the meditation. A typical meditation might go something like this (the meditator in this case has chosen the task of counting to three repeatedly):

> *One...two...this isn't so hard...one...two...three...one... I'm not having many thoughts at all... oh, oh, I just had a thought...that was another one...two...my nose itches...one... I wonder if it's okay to scratch it...darn, there was another thought. I've got to try harder...one...two...three... one...two... I was judging myself pretty harshly. I'm not supposed to do that...one...two...three... one... I'm hungry...wonder what I'll cook tonight...one...two...three... I'm having way too many thoughts... I'll never get this right...one...two...now don't judge...one...two...three... one....*

Each time this meditator realizes that his mind has drifted to other thoughts, he chooses instead to dwell on the original object of his attention. By repeating this one moment of awareness, a moment that consists of noticing the thought and then refocusing the attention, over time a number of surprising realizations can become apparent:

- It is impossible to worry, fear, or hate when your mind is thinking about something other than the object of these emotions.

- It isn't necessary to think about everything that pops into your head. You have the ability to choose which thoughts you will think about.

- The seemingly diverse contents of your mind really can fit into a few simple categories: grudging thoughts, fearful thoughts, angry thoughts, wanting thoughts, planning thoughts, memories, and so on.

- You act in certain ways because you have certain thoughts that over your lifetime have become habitual. Habitual patterns of thought and perception will begin to lose their influence over your life once you become aware of them.

- Emotions, aside from the thoughts and pictures in your mind, consist entirely of physical sensations in your body.

- Even the strongest emotion will become manageable if you concentrate on the sensations in your body and not the content of the thought that produced the emotion.

- Thoughts and emotions are not permanent. They pass into and out of your body and mind. They need not leave a trace.

- When you are awake to what is happening right now and open to what is, the extreme highs and extreme lows of your emotional response to life will disappear. You will live life with equanimity.

In 1968, Dr. Herbert Benson and his colleagues at Harvard Medical School decided to put meditation to the test. Volunteer practitioners of transcendental meditation were tested to see if meditation really could counter the physiological effects of stress. Benson scientifically proved that during meditation, the following physiological effects were observed:

1. Heartbeat and breathing rates slow down.

2. Oxygen consumption falls by 20 percent.

3. Blood lactate levels drop. (This level rises with stress and fatigue.)

4. Skin resistance to electrical current, a sign of relaxation, increases fourfold.

5. EEG ratings of brain-wave patterns indicate increased alpha activity, another sign of relaxation.

Benson (1997) went on to prove that any meditation practice could duplicate these physiological changes as long as the following four factors were present:

1. A relatively quiet environment

2. A mental device that provides a constant stimulus

3. A comfortable position

4. A passive attitude

With regular meditation, you will feel more focused and calmer in your life, more capable of making new choices in the moment, and less prone to engage in struggle and reactive responses.

Symptom-Relief Effectiveness

Meditation has been used successfully in the treatment and prevention of high blood pressure, heart disease, migraine headaches, and autoimmune diseases such as diabetes and arthritis. It has proved helpful in curtailing obsessive thinking, anxiety, depression, and hostility.

Time to Master

The benefits of meditation increase with practice. Levels of relaxation deepen. Attention becomes steadier. You become more adept at living in the present moment. For these three reasons, it is important to meditate regularly.

Instructions

The following sections address some important aspects of meditation: the importance of correct posture, the need to center yourself, and the amount of time to spend on the practice.

Establishing Your Posture

1. From the following, select a position that is comfortable for you:

   • In a chair with your knees comfortably apart, legs uncrossed, and hands resting in your lap.

   • Tailor fashion (cross-legged) on the floor. This position is most comfortable and stable when a cushion is placed under your buttocks so that both knees touch the floor.

   • On your knees with your big toes touching and your heels pointed outward so that your buttocks rest on the soles of your feet. Again, if you place a cushion between your feet for your buttocks to rest on, you will be able to hold the position for a much longer period of time (Japanese fashion).

2. Sit with your back straight (but not ramrod rigid) and let the weight of your head rest directly on your spinal column. This can be accomplished by pulling in your chin slightly. Allow the small of your back to arch.

3. Rock briefly from side to side, then from front to back, and establish the point at which your upper torso feels balanced on your hips.

4. Close your mouth and breathe through your nose. Place your tongue on the roof of your mouth.

Establishing Your Posture

Tailor fashion   Japanese fashion

Centering Yourself

Being centered means deliberately keeping an area of calmness within yourself by conscious thought no matter how intensely your emotions might be churning. For that reason, being centered is sometimes compared to being the eye in the center of a hurricane. The following are three steps to centering yourself:

Grounding

Close your eyes and focus on the place where your body touches the cushion or chair. What are the sensations there? Next, notice the places where your body touches itself. Are your hands crossed? Are your legs crossed? Pay attention to the sensation at these places of contact. Finally, focus on the way your body fills the space around you. Does it take up a lot of space or a small amount? Can you feel the boundary between your body and space? Notice the feelings there.

Breathing

With your eyes closed, take several deep breaths and notice the quality of your breathing. Is it fast or slow? Deep or shallow? Notice where your breath rests in your body. Is it up high in your chest? Is it in the midsection around your stomach? Down low in your belly? Try moving your breath from one area to the other. Breathe into your upper chest, then into your stomach, and then drop your breath into your lower belly. Feel your abdomen expand and contract as the air goes in and out. Notice how the upper chest and stomach areas seem almost still. This *dropped breath* is the most relaxing stance to meditate from. However, if you have difficulty taking deep belly breaths, don't worry. Your breath will drop of its own accord as you become more practiced in meditation.

Attitude

Maintaining a passive attitude during meditation is perhaps the most important element in eliciting relaxation. It is important to realize that, especially as a beginner, you will have many thoughts and relatively few moments of clear concentration. This is natural and to be expected. Realize that your thoughts are not really interruptions but are an integral part of meditation. Without thoughts arising, you would not be able to develop the ability to let them go.

A passive attitude includes a lack of concern about whether you are doing things correctly, whether you are accomplishing any goals, or whether this meditation is right for you. Sit with the attitude of "I'm going to put in my time here, just sitting, and whatever happens is exactly what should happen."

A Word About Time

In general, any amount of time spent in meditation is more relaxing than not meditating at all. When you first begin to practice, maintain the meditation for only as long as is comfortable even if this is just for five minutes a day. If you feel that you are forcing yourself to sit, you may develop an aversion to practicing meditation at all. As you progress in your practice and meditation becomes easier, you will find yourself wanting to extend your time. In terms of relaxation, twenty to thirty minutes once or twice a day is sufficient.

Exercises

The following meditation exercises are divided into four types:

- Type 1 is a group of three basic meditations. Try each one a few times, and settle on the one you like best. Practice it regularly, at least once a day.

- Type 2 introduces several mindfulness exercises. You don't have to go off by yourself and sit in silence in order to concentrate and build mindfulness. These exercises can be practiced anywhere and can be helpful in calming your body as it responds to stress throughout the day.

- Type 3 helps you develop mindfulness techniques to cope with pain or discomfort. In real life you may often find yourself in the presence of minor pain, annoyances, or disappointments, all of which can cause you to tense up. By practicing feeling relaxed in response to small irritations while you meditate, you will become more adept at handling life's larger irritations when they occur.

- Type 4 teaches you how to let go of obsessive thoughts and feelings that make it difficult to relax because your mind wants to hold on to an idea or emotion that you experienced at an earlier time.

Type 1: Three Basic Meditations

Mantra Meditation

The mantra meditation is the most common form of meditation throughout the world. Before you begin, select a word or syllable that pleases you. Perhaps there's a word that has special meaning for you. Or you may use nonsense syllables, the sound of which you find pleasant. Benson recommends using the word "one." Many meditators prefer the mantra "om."

1. Find your comfortable posture and center yourself. Take several deep breaths.

2. Chant your mantra silently to yourself. Say the word or syllables over and over within your mind. When your thought strays, note it and then bring your attention back to your mantra. If you notice any sensations in your body, note the feeling; then return to the repetition of your own special word. You needn't force it. Let your mantra find its own rhythm as you repeat it over and over again.

3. If you have the opportunity, you may want to try chanting your mantra aloud. Let the sound of your voice fill you as you relax. Notice whether the sensations in your body are different from those you felt when you chanted silently. Which is more relaxing?

4. Remember that meditation is to be practiced with awareness. You may find that the repetition of a mantra, especially when repeated silently, can easily become mechanical. When this happens, you may have the sense that an inner voice is repeating your mantra while you are actually lost in thought or rapidly approaching sleep. Try to stay aware of each repetition of each syllable.

Sitting Meditation

The simplest way to begin meditation is by focusing on your breath.

1. Choose a comfortable sitting posture.

2. Bring your attention to the gentle rise and fall of your breath. Like ocean waves coming in to the shore and going out, your breath is always there. You can focus on your inhale and exhale, the sensations of your breath entering your nose or mouth, or the sensations of your breath filling your lungs and diaphragm.

3. Whenever your mind wanders, gently bring your attention back to focus on your breath. Let your breath be your anchor to this present moment.

4. When you find yourself becoming distracted by thoughts, simply notice and acknowledge them.

5. One way to work with thoughts is to name them as you notice them. If you notice you are worrying, silently say to yourself, *Worry, worry, there is worry.* You can name *planning, reminiscing, longing, thinking,* or whatever it is in just the same way: label it and move on. This will help you to stop identifying yourself with your thoughts and to learn how to let go to create more spaciousness and peace.

This meditation can take between twenty and thirty minutes to do. With practice, you will become able to rest your attention on your breath more effortlessly and to let go of your thoughts more easily.

Breath-Counting Meditation

An alternative form of sitting meditation is the use of counting with the rhythm of the breath. Following the gentle ins and outs of the breath creates a sense of peace and restfulness.

1. Find your posture and center yourself. Take several deep breaths. Either close your eyes or fix them on a spot on the floor about four feet in front of you. Your eyes may be focused or not.

2. Take deep but not forced belly breaths. As you do, focus your attention on each part of the breath: the inhale, the turn (the point at which you stop inhaling and start exhaling), the exhale, the pause (between the exhale and inhale), the turn (the point at which you start to inhale), the inhale, and so on. Pay careful attention to the pause. What are the sensations in your body as you pause between breaths?

3. As you exhale, say "one." Continue counting each exhale: "two…three…four." Then begin again with "one." If you lose count, simply start over.

4. When you discover that your mind has slipped into thought, note this and then gently return to the counting of your breath.

5. If a particular sensation in your body catches your attention, focus on the sensation until it recedes. Then return your attention to the inhale and the exhale and the counting of your breath.

Type 2: Mindfulness and Present-Moment Awareness

Much of our stress comes from thinking about the past or worrying about the future. When you live in the present moment and your attention is focused on what you are doing right now, there is no room for anything else to enter—including regrets, anticipation of rejection or failure, or anything else that might be stressful.

In the meditative state, your attention is focused on the object of meditation, whether that's the inhale, the exhale, or the mantra that quiets the mind and allows you to be more in the present moment. When thoughts of past or future, desires or aversions, or anything else arise, you note this and then turn your awareness gently back to the present. This concentration on the here and now allows your body and mind to enter a state of relaxation.

Mindfulness meditation is a form of meditation that offers both deep relaxation and insight. It cultivates a way of being in a harmonious relationship with what is, whether that's nagging or obsessive thoughts, uncomfortable feelings, external stressors, or physical discomfort. By fully opening to what is present in your internal experience and not resisting or pushing it away, you can cultivate a deep acceptance and ability to rest more fully in the present moment. In the beginning stages of mindfulness practice, present-moment awareness is usually cultivated by focusing on the breath. Beginning practices can also include focusing on sounds, feelings, or body sensations. The body scanning exercises in chapter 2 or a mindful-movement discipline such as yoga, tai chi, or qi gong can also help cultivate mindfulness.

Whatever your focus of attention, a gentle, nonjudgmental, and embracing attitude should be used to encounter what arises during your course of meditation. The stories you tell yourself about what you notice and the reactivity to *what is* creates your suffering or pain. Use a bare-bones (that is, a primary or low-level) attention to simply notice wherever your attention goes during meditation, let go of it without judgment, and return to the object of focus that you've chosen. If you find yourself creating a story about it, such as, *Oh my left knee is really hurting, it will never stop, it's going to get worse*…simply notice the thought or story and return back to your breath without getting caught up in the content of your thoughts. Continue this process throughout the sitting period. Meditating in this way actually trains you to encounter stressors in your life, whether internal or external, in a similar fashion. When you encounter stressors, catch yourself before going into a habitual reaction that leads to suffering—rather than getting stuck in reactivity, breathe, pause, and make new choices about how to respond. Make choices that bring you healthier thinking, relaxation, insight, health, connection with others, and more love.

Eating Meditation

You eat every day, but how often do you really pay attention to what you are eating while you are eating it? Do you usually eat with other people? In front of the TV? While reading a book? Can you usually finish a three-course meal in ten minutes or even less time?

The following is a conscious-eating meditation. Try it someplace where it is unlikely anyone will want to come over and eat with you. For the sake of this example, the food in question is a cheese sandwich.

1. Sit down in front of your food and take several deep breaths. Note the food's color, shape, and texture. Does it seem appealing to you? Can you barely restrain yourself from gobbling it up? Whatever you're feeling, notice it.

2. Be aware of your intention to begin eating. Move your hand slowly toward the sandwich. As you do this, make a quiet mental note of the action. You may say to yourself, *Reaching…reaching…reaching.* By labeling your actions, you are more likely to keep in mind your purpose—to stay aware. As you pick up the sandwich, notice that you are *lifting…lifting…lifting.*

3. Watch your hand move the sandwich closer to your mouth. When it nears your mouth, take a moment to smell the food. What smells do you recognize? Can you smell the mayonnaise? How is your body reacting to the smell? Is your mouth watering? Notice the sensation of your body desiring food.

4. As you take your first bite, feel your teeth penetrate the bread. When the bite is complete, how is the food positioned in your mouth? How does your tongue position the food so that it's between your teeth? Begin chewing slowly. What are the sensations in your teeth? Your tongue? How does your tongue move when you chew? What tastes are you experiencing? The tomato? The cheese? What part of your tongue experiences the taste? Where is your arm? Did you put it back on the table? If so, did you notice the motion?

5. When you swallow, try to be aware of how the muscles in your esophagus contract and relax as they push the food to your stomach. Where is the food when you have finished swallowing? Can you feel the sensations in your stomach? Where is your stomach? What size is it? Is it empty, full, or somewhere in between?

6. As you continue to eat your sandwich, try to stay aware of as many sensations as you can. Silently label each movement if this helps. Try eating with the hand you don't normally use, because the awkwardness may serve as a reminder to pay attention. As with your basic meditation, when thoughts arise, notice them and then return your attention to your food.

Walking Meditation

Most people cover miles in the course of their daily routines. This makes walking a good opportunity to practice mindfulness. Focus on the act of walking much the same way as you focus on your breath in sitting meditation. You can do the walking meditation either indoors or outdoors.

1. Stand up and relax your abdominal muscles. Take several deep belly breaths. Feel your abdomen expand and contract with each breath. Begin walking. As you practice this exercise, try to continue breathing from this relaxed stance. Mentally repeat the word "in" with each inhalation and "out" with each exhalation as you walk.

2. Try to arrange it so that one of your feet touches the ground at the beginning of each *in* breath and each *out* breath, without forcing your breathing too much. Now, see how many steps seem natural to take during each inhalation and each exhalation.

3. As with all meditations, when thoughts or images interrupt your focus, make a mental note of this and then return to your walking and breathing.

4. Pay attention to the sensations of walking. Concentrate on your feet and lower legs. Notice which muscles contract and which relax as you lift your legs up and down. Which part of your foot touches the ground first? Pay attention to how your weight shifts from one foot to the other. What are the feelings in your knees as they bend and straighten? And, while you're at it, pay attention to the ground. What is its texture? Is it hard or soft? Notice any cracks or stones. How does the sensation of walking on grass differ from that of walking on a sidewalk? Catch your thoughts, let them go, and return to your awareness of the details of your present moment.

An alternative way to practice the walking meditation is to count your steps in time with your breathing as you walk. If you are taking three steps during each inhalation and exhalation, mentally say to yourself, *In…two…three. Out…two…three. In…two…three…*and so on. Your *in* breaths may be longer or shorter than your *out* breaths and therefore may accommodate either more or fewer steps. Or your step count may vary from breath to breath. Just pay attention and readjust your walking to the ins and outs of your breathing, as needed.

Seeing Meditation

You can gaze meditatively at something during a meeting, on a bus, or in a waiting room. This is a wonderfully inconspicuous meditation practice that can be done anywhere.

1. Find an object within your line of vision that you might want to fix your eyes on. Take several belly breaths as you glue your eyes to the object. Let it capture your interest, as though it were the only object in the vicinity. Try not to judge what you are seeing, or have any thoughts about it at all. See if you can have the experience of just seeing. When thoughts arise, note them and then return your focus to the object.

2. Try practicing this exercise with different types of objects. Here are a few suggestions:

    •   Concrete objects—objects with a definite size and shape that are usually stationary

    •   Natural objects—such as clouds, sand, a pile of dry leaves, the ocean, and so on

    •   Vastness—any large, uniform surface, such as a wall or a finely patterned rug

    •   Moving objects—a crowd of people, cars on a busy street, and so on. With objects of this nature, don't follow individual shapes with your eyes. Instead, fix your eyes on a point in space and let the movement pass in front of your field of vision.

Any simple activity can become a meditation when you try to continuously focus your attention on it. Another good mindfulness exercise is to choose an activity you do every day, preferably a short one, and then concentrate on every action and every sensation involved in that activity. Use the type of mental notation discussed earlier, under Eating Meditation, if that helps.

You could practice concentrating when you shave, brush your teeth, wash dishes, fold clothes, or pull weeds. As thoughts occur, note them, and then go back to the task with renewed concentration. While engaged in this activity, it is often helpful to use your nondominant hand (though you might not want to do this while shaving). The resulting awkwardness will serve as a constant reminder that you want to concentrate on what you are doing.

Type 3: Mindfulness of Pain or Discomfort

As a rule, most people respond to pain, irritation, or any physical discomfort by trying to build a solid wall of tightness around it, attempting to block off the feeling or to avoid it entirely. However, the more you resist pain, the more it hurts. And the more it hurts, the more you will try to resist it. This vicious cycle produces one big knot of pain and resistance that is extremely difficult to untie.

An alternative way to deal with pain is to learn to soften around it. This means you first acknowledge the pain's presence and then simply allow yourself to experience both physically and mentally whatever it is that hurts. Be your own good nurse, hold your own hand, tell yourself it's all right, and then sit with yourself compassionately as you experience sensations of discomfort.

When you open to an irritation, you consciously relax your tense, clenched muscles around the spot that hurts. You focus on the hurting itself, without all the tightness you tend to add to it.

Softening also means that you notice but disregard your thoughts about how awful the discomfort is, how you have to move, how you have to scratch, how you can't stand it, and so on. Softening is like working the hard lumps out of a mound of clay so that you can feel a tiny pearl in the center. It's like removing screens placed around a candle flame so that you can see it clearly. It's like thawing out the frozen core of a large piece of meat so that you can remove the bone. It's like cleaning layers of grime off the outside of a window so that you can see what's inside more clearly.

The following exercise introduces minor irritations into your basic meditation. By practicing with small irritations in a safe setting, you can begin to understand the process of softening.

Don't Move

1. Find your posture and center yourself. Take several deep breaths.

2. Make an agreement with yourself that for a preset period of time you will not move. Then begin your basic meditation.

3. As time passes, you may find yourself moving your head or shifting in your seat without realizing it. This is fine. Note the movement and return to your meditation. After a while you will be able to notice your intention to move a part of your body before you actually move it.

4. Once you are able to identify your intention to move, try to focus on what exactly your desire is. Do you want to squirm around in your chair? Stretch your back muscles? Maybe you have an itch or an ant is crawling across your foot. Try to precisely identify the uncomfortable sensation. Remember, don't move.

5. As you focus on the discomfort, try to soften around it. If muscle groups are tightening, try to relax them. Check these muscle groups often, because they will not want to stay relaxed. Where is your breath? Is it high in your chest? If so, try to drop it into your belly. Focus on the sensation of discomfort. What is the feeling here? Stay with it for a while.

6. When time is up, move your body slowly to the position you've been wanting to sit in. Focus on the sensations. Is the relief immediate? Is the relief gradual? In what way does your body feel better? Is there any tension? If so, release it.

Any irritating sound or sensation can be used as a focal point for meditation. Focusing on your body's minor aches or the sound of a lawn mower or a dog barking can teach you how your body responds to life's irritations. Once you realize this, you can begin to learn how to soften around such irritations.

Type 4: Letting Go of Thoughts

This highly structured exercise is found in many cultures in one form or another. In it, you passively observe the flow of your thoughts, feelings, and perceptions, one after another, without being concerned with their meaning or their relationship to one another. This will allow you to see what's on your mind and then let it go.

Go with the Flow

1. Find your posture and center yourself. Take several deep breaths.

2. Close your eyes and imagine yourself sitting at the bottom of a deep pool of water. When you have a thought, feeling, or perception, see it as a bubble and let it rise away from you and disappear. When it's gone, wait for the next one to appear, and repeat the process. Don't think about the contents of the bubble. Just observe it. Sometimes the same bubble may come up many times, or several bubbles will seem related to each other, or the bubbles may be empty. That's okay. Don't allow yourself to be concerned with these thoughts. Just watch them pass in front of your mind's eye.

3. If you feel uncomfortable imagining being underwater, imagine that you are sitting on the bank of a river, watching a leaf drift slowly downstream. Imagine one thought, feeling, or perception as the leaf, and then let it drift out of sight. Return to gazing at the river, waiting for the next leaf to float by with a new thought. Or, if you prefer, you can imagine your thoughts rising in puffs of smoke from a campfire.

Special Considerations

- It is not necessary to feel as though you are relaxing while you meditate for you to actually become relaxed. You may feel as though you are thinking thousands of thoughts and are very restless. However, when you open your eyes at the end of your meditation, you will realize you feel much more relaxed than you did before you began meditating.

- As your mind quiets with meditation, old or hidden pain can arise from your subconscious. If you find that when you meditate you suddenly feel angry, depressed, or frightened, try to gently allow yourself to experience the feeling without resistance and let go of the temptation to make sense out of your feelings. If you feel the need, talk to a friend, counselor, or meditation teacher.

- You may hear or read about ideal conditions for meditation: for example, that you should meditate only in a quiet place, only two hours after you've eaten, or only in a position that you can hold comfortably for twenty minutes, and so on. Yes, these are ideal conditions, but life is seldom ideal. If the place isn't absolutely quiet or if the only time you have to meditate is right after lunch, don't let these small obstacles keep you from meditating. If you find yourself being particularly bothered by noises or the rumblings of a full stomach, simply incorporate the annoying sensation in with the object of your meditation.

- If you adopt a daily sitting practice, you may find there are stretches of time during which you will not want to meditate. Don't expect that your desire to meditate will grow constantly with your practice. If you feel discouraged, be gentle with yourself and try to work creatively on ways to make your practice more comfortable. Know that these periods of discouragement will go away by themselves in time. Here are two things you can do to help maintain a schedule: Pick a regular time of the day to meditate and honor it as you would any other appointment. Find a group to meditate with—the value of finding such a group cannot be overstated.

The practice of meditation can bring focus, insight, and a sense of renewal to your life. Give yourself the gift of meditation and all of its benefits.

Further Reading

Benson, H. 1997. *Timeless Healing: The Power of Biology and Belief.* Reprint ed. New York: Scribner.

Brantley, J. 2007. *Calming Your Anxious Mind: How Mindfulness and Compassion Can Free You from Anxiety, Fear, and Panic.* 2nd ed. Oakland, CA: New Harbinger Publications.

Goldstein, J. 1987. *The Experience of Insight.* Reissue ed. Boston: Shambhala Publications.

Goldstein, J., and J. Kornfield. 1995. *The Path of Insight Meditation.* Boston: Shambhala Publications.

————. 2001. *Seeking the Heart of Wisdom.* Reprint ed. Boston: Shambhala Publications.

Hewitt, J. 1990. *The Complete Yoga Book.* Reissue ed. New York: Schocken Books.

Kabat-Zinn, Jon. 1994. *Wherever You Go, There You Are: Mindfulness Meditation in Everyday Life.* New York: Hyperion.

————. 2005. *Coming to Our Senses: Healing Ourselves and the World Through Mindfulness.* New York: Hyperion.

————. 2013. *Full Catastrophe Living: Using the Wisdom of Your Body and Mind to Face Stress, Pain, and Illness.* Revised and updated ed. New York: Bantam Books.

Kornfield, J. 1993. *A Path with Heart: A Guide Through the Perils and Promises of Spiritual Life.* New York: Bantam Books.

LeShan, L. 1999. *How to Meditate.* New York: Little, Brown and Company.

Nhat Hahn, Thich. 1992. *Peace Is Every Step: The Path of Mindfulness in Everyday Life.* New York: Bantam Books.

————. 1999. *The Miracle of Mindfulness.* Boston: Beacon Press.

————. 2005. *Being Peace.* 2nd ed. Berkeley, CA: Parallax Press.

Recordings

Goleman, D. 1989. *The Art of Meditation* (Audio CD). New York: Holzbrink.

Kabat-Zinn, Jon. 2005. *Guided Mindfulness Meditation* (Audio CD). Louisville, CO: Sounds True.

————. 2006. *Mindfulness for Beginners* (Audio CD). Louisville, CO: Sounds True.

Nhat Hanh, Thich. 2005. *Touching Peace* (Audio CD). Berkeley, CA: Parallax Press.

CHAPTER 6

Visualization

In this chapter you will learn to:

- Use your imagination to relax

- Manage stress-related conditions

- Create a safe and relaxing place in your mind

Background

You can significantly reduce stress with an enormously powerful force: your imagination. The practice of positive thinking for the treatment of physical symptoms was popularized by Emil Coué, a French pharmacist, at the turn of the nineteenth century. He believed that the power of the imagination far exceeds that of the will. It's hard to will yourself into a relaxed state, but you can imagine relaxation spreading through your body, and you can visualize yourself in a safe and beautiful refuge. Coué asserted that all of your thoughts become reality—you are what you think you are. For example, if you think sad thoughts, you feel unhappy. If you think anxious thoughts, you become tense.

In order to overcome the feeling of unhappiness or tension, you can refocus your mind on positive, healing images. When you predict that you are going to be lonely and miserable, your prediction will probably come true, because your negative thoughts will be reflected in your asocial behavior. A woman who predicts that she will get a stomachache when her boss yells at her is likely to have her thoughts take a somatic form. Coué found that organic diseases such as fibrous tumors, tuberculosis, hemorrhages, and constipation are often worsened when you focus on them. His patients were recommended to say aloud, upon awakening, at least twenty times a day, the now-famous phrase "Every day in every way I am getting better and better."

Coué also encouraged his patients to get into a comfortable, relaxed position when retiring, and then to close their eyes and practice general relaxation of all their muscles. As they started to doze off in the stage of semiconsciousness, he suggested that they introduce into their minds any desired idea, for example, "I am going to be relaxed tomorrow." Coué understood that this is a way of bridging your conscious and unconscious minds and allowing your unconscious to make a wish come true.

In the twentieth century, Carl Jung used a technique for healing that he referred to as "active imagination." He instructed his patients to meditate without any goal or program in mind. Images would come to consciousness that the patient was to observe and experience without interference. Later, if desired, the patient could actually communicate with the images by asking them questions or talking to them. Jung used active imagination to help individuals appreciate their rich inner life and learn to draw on its healing power in times of stress. Jungian and gestalt therapists have since devised several stress reduction techniques using the intuitive, imaginative part of the mind.

Today, visualization is practiced and studied in cancer and pain centers throughout the country. Stephanie Matthews and O. Carl Simonton, who pioneered the use of visualization with cancer patients, wrote *Getting Well Again* in 1978. Two other visualization scientists, therapists, and writers are Jeanne Achterberg, who wrote *Imagery in Healing* in 1985, and Connecticut surgeon and Yale professor Bernie S. Siegel, who wrote *Love, Medicine, and Miracles* in 1986.

Shakti Gawain, author of *Creative Visualization* (2016) and *Living in the Light* (1993), states that visualization is a form of energy that creates life and life's happenings. Everything is energy and our mind creates our world, much as a movie projector casts a world upon a blank screen.

Symptom-Relief Effectiveness

Visualization is effective in treating many stress-related and physical illnesses, including headaches, muscle spasms, chronic pain, and general or situation-specific anxiety. Visualization is used to prepare patients for surgery, to boost the effects of chemotherapy, to increase focus in sports competition, and to enhance well-being.

Time to Master

Symptom relief can be immediate or may take up to several weeks of practice.

Instructions

Types of Visualization

Everybody visualizes. Daydreams, memories, and inner talk are all types of visualization. You can harness your visualizations and consciously employ them to better yourself and your life. *Visualizations* are mental sense impressions you create consciously to relax your body and relieve stress. There are three types of visualization for change: receptive visualization, programmed visualization, and guided visualization.

1. **Receptive visualization.** With this type, you relax, empty your mind, sketch an image of a scene, ask a question, and wait for a response. For example, you might imagine you are on a beach and the sea breeze is caressing your skin. You can hear and smell the sea. Then you might ask, *Why can't I relax?* And the response might surface into your consciousness, for example, *Because you can't say no to people,* or *Because you can't detach yourself from your husband's depression.*

2. **Programmed visualization.** Create an image, replete with sights, taste, sounds, and smells. Then, imagine a goal that you want to attain or a healing that you want to accelerate. For instance, Harriet used programmed visualization when she started running. For her first race, she visualized her race on that course daily. She would feel the pressure of running up a hill, the exhaustion after several miles, and the sprint to the finish line. When she finally ran that race, she set a state record for her age group that still holds.

3. **Guided visualization.** Again, visualize your scene in detail, but omit crucial elements. Then wait for your subconscious, or your inner guide, to supply the missing pieces in your puzzle. Jane imagines visiting a special place where she likes to relax. She constructs the smells, tastes, sounds, touch, and sights associated with the place, a forest clearing that she used to visit with the Girl Scouts. She sees herself roasting marshmallows over a campfire at twilight. (There are no mosquitoes.) She imagines her Girl Scout leader, someone she loves, and asks the leader how she can relax. Sometimes the Scout leader reminds her of songs she used to love and she tells Jane to sing them whenever she feels tense. Sometimes she reminds Jane of old jokes and old times that made Jane laugh, and she tells Jane that she needs to laugh more. Often the leader gives Jane a hug, to remind her that she is loved and that she needs to search for affirmations of that love.

Rules for Effective Visualization

1. Loosen your clothing, lie down in a quiet place, and softly close your eyes.

2. Scan your body, seeking tension in specific muscles. Relax those muscles as much as you can.

3. Form mental sense impressions. Involve all your senses: sight, hearing, smell, touch, and taste. For instance, imagine you are in the midst of a green forest with beautiful trees, vivid blue sky, and fluffy white clouds. Then add the sounds: wind in the trees, water running, birdcalls, and so on. Imagine you can hear pine needles crunching underfoot. Include the feel of the ground under your shoes, the smell of pine, and the taste of a grass stem or mountain spring water.

4. Use affirmations. Repeat short, positive statements that affirm your ability to relax now. Use the present tense and avoid negatives, such as "I am not tense," in favor of positive versions, such as "I am letting go of tension." Here are some other examples of affirmations: *Tension flows from my body. I can relax at will. I am in harmony with life. Peace is within me.*

5. Practice creating your visualization three times a day. Visualization practice is easiest when done in the morning and at night while you lie in bed. After some practice, you will be able to visualize while waiting in the doctor's office, at the service station, before going into a parent-teacher conference—even during an IRS audit.

Basic Tension and Relaxation Exercises

1. Eye Relaxation (Palming)

Place your palms directly over your closed eyes. Block out all light without putting too much pressure on your eyelids. Try to see the color black. You may see other colors or images, but focus on the color black. Use a mental image to remember the color black (black fur, black object in the room).

Continue this way for two to three minutes, thinking and focusing on black. Lower your hands and slowly open your eyes, gradually getting accustomed to the light. Experience the sense of relaxation in the muscles that control the opening and closing of your eyes.

2. Metaphorical Images

Lie down, close your eyes, and relax. Visualize an image for tension and then replace it with an image for relaxation. The best images are those you make up yourself. But to get you started, images for tension might include the following:

- the color red
- the screech of chalk on a blackboard
- the tension of a cable
- the scream of a siren in the night
- the glare of a searchlight
- the smell of ammonia
- the confinement of a dark tunnel
- the pounding of a jackhammer

These tension images during visualization can soften, expand, and fade, creating relaxation and harmony:

- The color red can fade to pale blue.

- The chalk can crumble into powder.

- The cable can slacken.

- The siren might soften to a whisper of a flute.

- The searchlight might fade into a soft rosy glow.

- The smell of ammonia might soften into the smell of lemon or a rose.

- The dark tunnel might open into a light, airy beach.

- The jackhammer can become the hands of a masseuse kneading your muscles.

As you scan your body, apply a tension image to a tense muscle. Allow it to develop into your relaxation image. For example, if your neck is tense, you may visualize a tightened vise. Imagine the vise opening as you say an affirmation such as *Relax* or *I can relax at will*.

End by reciting your affirmation. Speak to the specific tenseness as you apply your relaxation image. Observe what happens to your tension.

3. Creating Your Special Place

In creating your special place you will be making a refuge for relaxation and guidance. This place can be indoors or out. When structuring your place, follow these few guidelines:

- Allow a private entry into your place.

- Make it peaceful, comfortable, and safe.

- Fill your place with sensuous detail. Create a middle ground, foreground, and background.

- Allow room for an inner guide or other person to be there with you comfortably.

A special place might be at the end of a path that leads to a pond. Grass grows under your feet, the pond is about thirty yards away, and mountains are in the distance. You can feel the coolness of the air in this shady spot. The mockingbird is singing. The sun is bright on the pond. The honeysuckle's pungent odor attracts the bee buzzing over the flowers with their sweet nectar.

Or your special place might be a sparkling clean kitchen with cinnamon buns baking in the oven. Through the kitchen window you can see fields of yellow wheat. A window chime flutters in the breeze. At the table there's a cup of tea for your guest.

Try recording this exercise and playing it, or have a friend read it aloud to you slowly:

To go to your safe place, lie down and be totally comfortable. Close your eyes.... Walk slowly to a quiet place in your mind.... Your place can be inside or outside.... It needs to be peaceful and safe.... Picture yourself unloading your anxieties, your worries.... Notice the view in the distance.... What do you smell?... What do you hear?... Notice what is before you.... Reach out and touch it.... How does it feel?... Smell it.... Hear it.... Make the temperature comfortable.... Be safe here.... Look around for a special spot, a private spot.... Find the path to this place.... Feel the ground with your feet.... Look above you.... What do you see?... Hear?... Smell?... Walk down this path until you can enter your own quiet, comfortable, safe place.

You have arrived at your special place.... What is under your feet?... How does it feel?... Take several steps.... What do you see above you? What do you hear? Do you hear something else? Reach for and touch something.... What is its texture? Are there pens, paper, or paints nearby, or is there sand to draw in, clay to work? Go to them, handle them, smell them. These are your special tools, or tools for your inner guide to reveal ideas or feelings to you.... Look as far as you can see.... What do you see? What do you hear? What aromas do you notice?

Sit or lie in your special place.... Notice its smells, sounds, sights.... This is your place and nothing can harm you here.... If danger is here, expel it.... Spend three to five minutes realizing you are relaxed, safe, and comfortable.

Memorize this place's smells, tastes, sights, sounds.... You can come back and relax here whenever you want.... Leave by the same path or entrance.... Notice the ground, touch things near you.... Look far away and appreciate the view.... Remind yourself that this special place you created can be entered whenever you wish. Say an affirmation such as "I can relax here" or "This is my special place. I can come here whenever I wish."

Now open your eyes and spend a few seconds appreciating your relaxation.

4. Finding Your Inner Guide

Your inner guide is an imaginary person or animal that clarifies and instructs. This being is your link to your own inner wisdom and to your subconscious. Your inner guide can tell you how to relax and can clarify what is causing your stress. With practice, you can meet your inner guide in your special place whenever you want.

Perhaps you already have an inner guide, a deceased parent or another spiritual presence. If so, invite this person into your special place to show you how to relax.

Try this exercise after reading it all the way through first, or record it, or have a friend read it aloud to you.

Relax and follow the path to your special place, as you have been doing. Invite an inner guide to your place. Wait. Watch your guide's path. Notice a speck in the distance. Wait. Watch your guide's approach. Listen to the footfalls. Can you smell the guide's fragrance? As your guide gains shape and clarity, if you feel unsafe, send it away. Wait for other guides until you find one you like, even though its appearance may surprise you or seem odd.

When your guide is comfortable, ask questions. Wait for the answers. An answer may be a laugh, a saying, a feeling, a dream, a frown, or a purr. Ask your guide, "How can I relax? What is causing my tension?" When your guide answers, you will probably be surprised at the simplicity and clarity of its answers.

Before your guide leaves you, or immediately after, say your affirmation to yourself. Affirm your ability to relax with a simple "I can relax here" or "I can relax at will."

Do this exercise several times a day for at least seven days. By the seventh day, you will probably have found a guide and some answers.

One student who lost his mother and his house, and whose father is unable to care for him, uses his mother as his inner guide. He goes to her to relax, to seek guidance when pressure from his life and his peers feels overwhelming. She doesn't say much, but her presence and her look of approval or disapproval is often enough to calm him.

Another person's guide can create relaxation simply because of the emptying of the mind that occurs in her presence. Words are rarely spoken, but her guide's actions and silence guide her.

Each person's inner guide is different and instructs in a unique manner.

5. Listening to Music

Listening to music is one of the most common forms of relaxation. However, everyone gives their own meaning to music. It's important, therefore, that when you want to listen to music for the purpose of relaxation, you select music you find peaceful and soothing. If possible, make or buy a half-hour recording of uninterrupted relaxing music that you can play daily or whenever you decide to use music to relax. Note that the repetition of the same music that helped you relax in the past carries a positive association that is likely to be beneficial in the future.

To get the most out of your music session, find a half hour of uninterrupted time to be alone. Put on the music you have chosen, settle back in a comfortable position, and close your eyes. Mentally scan your body, noting areas of tension, pain, and relaxation. Be aware of your mood as you focus your attention on the music. Each time an unrelated thought enters your head, note it and then discard it, remembering your goal of focusing on the music and relaxing. Say an affirmation, such as *Relax* or *Music relaxes me*. When the music ends, allow your mind to scan your body again and become aware of how it feels. Does your body feel different than before you started listening to music? Is there any difference in your mood?

Special Considerations

1. If you have trouble receiving impressions from all of your senses, work on your strongest sense first. The others will improve in time.

2. Practice often—three times a day. And be patient; it takes time.

3. If making your own recording doesn't work, you might want to buy one. There are some listed at the end of this chapter.

4. Remember to laugh. Laughter reduces emotional and physical tension by producing an internal massage. Laughing stimulates your circulatory, respiratory, vascular, and nervous systems. When the internal spasms of laughter subside, the release of pressure reduces muscle tension and creates a feeling of well-being. In his book *Anatomy of an Illness* (2005), Norman Cousins describes how he used laughter to overcome a rare and painful illness. Laughter takes your attention off yourself and your situation. It provides you with the distance necessary to gain perspective on a situation that you may be taking too seriously.

Visualization can help you relax and can assist you in bringing focus and clarity to your life. When practiced on a regular basis, it will increase your sense of well-being.

Further Reading

Achterberg, J., B. Dossey, and L. Kolkmeier. 1994. *Rituals of Healing: Using Imagery for Health and Wellness.* New York: Bantam Books.

Coué, E. 2006. *Self-Mastery Through Conscious Autosuggestions.* Overland Park, KS: Digireads.

Cousins, N. 1990. *Head First: The Biology of Hope and the Healing Power of the Human Spirit.* New York: Penguin Books.

———. 2005. *Anatomy of an Illness.* 20th anniversary ed. New York: W. W. Norton & Company.

Epstein, G. 1989. *Healing Visualization: Creating Health Through Imagery.* Reissue ed. New York: Bantam Books.

Gawain, S. 1993. *Living in the Light: A Guide to Personal and Planetary Transformation.* New York: Bantam Books.

———. 2016. *Creative Visualization: Use the Power of Your Imagination to Create What You Want in Life.* 40th anniversary ed. New York: New World Library.

Klein, A. 1989. *The Healing Power of Humor.* Los Angeles: J. P. Tarcher.

———. 1998. *The Courage to Laugh.* Los Angeles: J. P. Tarcher.

Ornstein, R. 1996. *The Psychology of Consciousness.* 2nd revised ed. New York: Penguin.

Rossman, M. L. 2000. *Guided Imagery for Self-Healing.* 2nd ed. New York: H. J. Kramer.

Siegel, B. 1998. *Love, Medicine, and Miracles.* Reissue ed. New York: HarperCollins.

Simonton, O. C., S. Matthews-Simonton, and J. L. Creighton. 1992. *Getting Well Again.* Reissue ed. New York: Bantam Books.

Wells, V. 1990. *The Joy of Visualization: 75 Creative Ways to Enhance Your Life.* San Francisco: Chronicle Books.

Recordings

Fanning, P. 1992. *Visualization for Healing Injuries* (Audio CD). Oakland, CA: New Harbinger Publications.

Fanning, P., and M. McKay. 1992. *Visualization for Stress Reduction* (Audio CD). Oakland, CA: New Harbinger Publications.

Gawain, S. 2002. *Creative Visualization Meditations* (Audio CD). New York: New World Library Audio.

Miller, E. 2003. *Letting Go of Stress* (Audio CD). Nevada City, CA: Emmett Miller. http://www.drmiller.com.

CHAPTER 7

Applied Relaxation Training

In this chapter you will learn to:

- **Relax quickly in stressful situations**

Background

Applied relaxation training brings together a number of proven relaxation techniques, including some already covered in this book. The combined effect is both rapid and powerful, helping you reverse the effects of high stress in less than a minute. Because the program is progressive, you will be adding new features to the exercise over the course of several weeks, while taking away other features once they have become habitual. Eventually, you will be able to achieve deep relaxation in twenty to thirty seconds, quickly calming both your body and your mind when you encounter a stressful situation.

The Swedish physician L.G. Öst developed applied relaxation in the late 1980s. Öst worked with phobic patients who needed rapid and reliable methods to cut through the anxiety that struck when they encountered phobic situations. In addition to finding that the technique could achieve high rates of success even with severely phobic patients, Öst realized that applied relaxation could be helpful in a variety of life situations, from daily quarrels and frustrations to difficulty falling asleep at night.

In general, the program first teaches you to relax by using a physical relaxation process. You then progress to a conditioned relaxation response and, finally, learn to relax on command. You will also progress from practicing in a relaxed exercise setting to using the technique in real-life situations.

Symptom-Relief Effectiveness

Although applied relaxation was first developed to treat patients with phobias, it has a wide range of applications in other areas, including panic disorder, generalized anxiety disorder, headaches (tension, migraine, and mixed), back and joint pain, epilepsy in both children and adults, and tinnitus. In clinical practice, applied relaxation training has also proven useful for sleep-onset insomnia, for cardiac neurosis (being needlessly preoccupied with the possibility of heart attack and typically requiring repeated reassurances from a doctor), and for cancer patients with chemotherapy-induced nausea (Öst 1987). Öst found that almost everyone can learn applied relaxation and that 90 to 95 percent of the patients in his studies experienced benefits from the training.

Time to Master

You will notice some relaxation after just one or two sessions of applied relaxation training. Remember that this is a progressive program. Each new stage will help you relax more quickly and more deeply until you can relax at will in less than a minute. Don't rush yourself. You'll want to master each step of the program before moving on to the next step. Allow yourself one to two weeks, with two practice sessions a day, to feel comfortable with each step. If this sounds like a lot of time, keep in mind that your practice sessions can become the most refreshing part of your day.

Clinical applications of applied relaxation have ranged from an unusually quick two-week course for inpatients suffering from tinnitus to a fourteen-week program for inpatients with panic disorders (Öst 1987). A middle range is more usual; generally, you can expect to spend from five to eight weeks progressing through the program.

Instructions

Applied relaxation training involves learning five separate stages. Each stage builds on the one before it, so be sure to follow all five stages in their listed order.

1. Progressive Muscle Relaxation

Progressive muscle relaxation will help you recognize the difference between tension and relaxation in each of your major muscle groups. Surprising as it may sound, these distinctions are easy to overlook. Once you can really feel the difference between a tense muscle and a deeply relaxed one, you will be able to identify your chronic trouble spots and consciously rid them of their locked-in tension. You will also be able to bring your muscles to a deeper state of relaxation after you relax them than you could have if you hadn't tensed them first. Follow the instructions described under Basic Procedure in chapter 4. Give yourself one to two weeks to master the technique, with two fifteen-minute practice sessions per day. Your goal should be to relax your entire body in one fifteen-to twenty-minute session.

2. Release-Only Relaxation

Now that you've felt the difference between tensing and relaxing each muscle group, you're ready to move on to the next stage of applied relaxation training. As you might guess from its name, release-only relaxation cuts out the first step in progressive muscle relaxation: the tensing step. This means that you can cut the time down by half (or more) needed to achieve deep relaxation in each muscle group.

With practice, you'll find that mental focus alone is enough to drain your muscles of their tension, with no need for you to tense them first. Developing this skill depends on your ability to recognize the difference between clenched muscles and deeply relaxed ones. Be sure that you're comfortable with progressive muscle relaxation before beginning the following release-only instructions.

A. Sit in a comfortable chair with your arms at your sides and move around a bit until you're comfortable.

B. Begin to focus on your breathing. Breathe in deeply and feel the pure air fill your stomach, your lower chest, and your upper chest. Hold your breath for a moment as you sit up straighter…and then breathe out slowly through your mouth, feeling all your tension and worries blow out in a stream of air. After you've exhaled completely, relax your stomach and your chest. Continue to take full, calm, even breaths, noticing that you become more relaxed with each exhalation.

C. Now relax your forehead, smoothing out all the lines. Keep breathing deeply…and now relax your eyebrows. Just let all the tension melt away, all the way down to your jaw. Let it all go. Now let your lips separate, and relax your tongue. Breathe in and breathe out and relax your throat. Notice how peaceful and loose your entire face feels now.

D. Roll your head gently and feel your neck relax. Release your shoulders. Just let them drop all the way down. Your neck is loose, and your shoulders are heavy and low. Now let the relaxation travel down through your arms to your fingertips. Your arms are heavy and loose. Your lips are still separated because your jaw is relaxed too.

E. Breathe in deeply and feel your stomach expand and then your chest. Hold your breath for a moment and then breathe out slowly in a smooth stream through your mouth.

F. Let the feeling of relaxation spread to your stomach. Feel all the muscles in your abdomen release their tension as it assumes its natural shape. Relax your waist and relax your back. Continue to breathe deeply. Notice how loose and heavy the upper half of your body feels.

G. Now relax the lower half of your body. Feel your buttocks sink into the chair. Relax your thighs. Relax your knees. Feel the relaxation travel through your calves to your ankles, to the bottoms of your feet, all the way down to the tips of your toes. Your feet feel warm and heavy on the floor in front of you. With each breath, feel the relaxation deepen.

H. Now scan your body for tension as you continue to breathe. Your legs are relaxed. Your back is relaxed. Your shoulders and arms are relaxed. Your face is relaxed. There's only a feeling of peace and warmth and relaxation.

I. If any muscle felt hard to relax, turn your attention to it now. Is it your back? Your shoulders? Your thighs? Your jaw? Tune in to the muscle, and now tense it. Hold it tighter and release. Feel it join the rest of your body in a deep, deep relaxation.

The directions for release-only relaxation may seem simpler than those for progressive muscle relaxation, but the tasks involved are actually a bit more complex. Be certain that you drain all of the tension out of each muscle that you focus on. Don't let the tension creep back in as you turn your attention to different muscles. When you stand up after a session of release-only relaxation, you should feel at least as relaxed as you did after a session of progressive muscle relaxation.

Of course, you don't want to stress yourself by forcing and pushing yourself through a set of strict directions. Allow your body to relax rather than forcing it. If you have trouble with a particular step, take a deep breath and try it again—or skip it. Let negative, critical thoughts blow away with each breath, and hold onto the feeling of success and deepening peace.

Allow yourself one to two weeks with two practice sessions a day to master release-only relaxation. When you can relax your entire body in one five- to seven-minute session, you're ready to move on to step 3.

3. Cue-Controlled Relaxation

Cue-controlled relaxation reduces the time you need to relax even further—down to two or three minutes in most cases. In this stage, you will focus on your breathing and condition yourself to relax exactly when you tell yourself to relax. The instructions will help you build an association between a cue—for example, the command "relax"—and true muscle relaxation. Be sure that you are comfortable with release-only relaxation before you begin to work with cue-controlled relaxation.

A. Make yourself comfortable in your chair, with your arms on your lap and your feet flat on the ground. Take a deep breath and hold it for a moment. Concentrate on blowing the worries of the day far, far away as you release the air from your mouth in a smooth stream. Empty your lungs as you feel your stomach and your chest relax.

B. Now begin to relax yourself, from your forehead all the way down to your toes, using the release-only technique. See if you can relax yourself completely in thirty seconds. If you need more time, that's fine.

C. You feel peaceful and at ease now. Your stomach and chest are moving in and out with slow, even breaths. With each breath, the feeling of relaxation deepens.

D. Continue to breathe deeply and regularly, saying *breathe in* to yourself as you inhale and *relax* as you exhale.

Breathe in…relax…

Breathe in…relax…

Breathe in…relax…

Breathe in…relax…

Breathe in…relax…

Feel each breath bring peace and calm in and float worry and tension out.

E. Continue this way for several minutes now, saying these words to yourself—*breathe in* and *relax*—while you breathe. Focus all your attention on the words in your head and on the process of breathing. Feel your muscles relax more and more deeply with each breath. Let the word "relax" crowd every other thought from your mind. Close your eyes if you can, to deepen your focus.

F. Now listen to the words again as you continue to breathe in…and relax.

Breathe in…relax…

Breathe in…relax…

Breathe in…relax…

Breathe in…relax…

Breathe in…relax…

G. Continue to breathe, saying these words in your head, for a few more minutes. Now, feel each breath bring peace and calm in and float worry and tension out.

H. If you have time, repeat the entire process of cue-controlled relaxation after a recovery period of between ten and fifteen minutes.

Practice cue-controlled relaxation twice a day as you did with the earlier practices.

After each session, you may want to make a note of the amount of time you needed to relax and how deeply relaxed you became. Most people find that the actual time required to relax at this stage is shorter than they imagine. Aim to relax completely within two to three minutes using cue-controlled relaxation before moving on to rapid relaxation.

4. Rapid Relaxation

Rapid relaxation can bring the time you need to relax down to thirty seconds. Being able to relax that quickly can mean real relief during stressful situations. It's a good idea to practice rapid relaxation many times a day as you move through different activities and states of mind.

In rapid relaxation, you will pick a special relaxation cue. Choose something that you see regularly throughout the day, such as your watch or a certain clock or the picture you pass as you walk down the hall to the bathroom. If you can, mark that special cue with a piece of colored tape while you're practicing this technique.

When you're ready to begin, look at your special cue. Breathe in and relax. Breathe in and relax. Continue to look at your cue and think *relax*. Breathe in and relax. You are breathing deeply and evenly, and you continue to think *relax* each time you exhale. Let the relaxation spread throughout your body. Scan your body for tension, and relax as much as possible in every muscle that isn't needed for whatever activity you are currently doing.

Every time you look at your cue throughout the day, go through these three simple steps:

A. Take two or three deep, even breaths, exhaling slowly through your mouth.

B. Think *relax* each time you exhale, as you continue to breathe deeply.

C. Scan your body for any tension. Focus on those muscles that need to relax and empty them of tension.

Try to use your relaxation cue fifteen times a day to relax quickly in natural, nonstressful situations. This will instill the habit of checking yourself for tension and moving back to a state of deep relaxation throughout the day. After your first few days of practice, you may want to change the color of the tape on your relaxation cue—or even change the cue altogether. This will keep the idea of relaxation fresh in your mind. Finally, see if you can use rapid relaxation to calm yourself during one or two particularly stressful moments of the day. (The final stage of applied relaxation will help you refine this ability, but it's a good idea to open yourself up early to the idea of relaxation during a crisis.)

When you feel comfortable with rapid relaxation and are able to achieve a state of deep relaxation in twenty to thirty seconds many times during the day, you are ready to move on to the final stage of applied relaxation training.

5. Applied Relaxation

Applied relaxation involves relaxing quickly in the face of anxiety-provoking situations. You will use the same techniques that you practiced in rapid relaxation, beginning your deep breathing the moment you notice a stress reaction setting in.

If you're unsure of your body's particular stress warning signs—such as rapid breathing, sweating, or an increased heart rate—turn to the body scanning exercises in chapter 2. The earlier you can identify the physiological signs that accompany stress, the more effectively you will be able to cut in on a stress reaction before it builds.

As soon as you note a sign of stress—if you catch your breath, feel your heart leap, or feel a flush of heat—begin your three steps:

A. Take two to three deep, even breaths.

B. Think these calming words to yourself as you continue to breathe deeply:

   Breathe in…relax…

   Breathe in…relax…

   Breathe in…relax…

   If you prefer, you need only hear yourself think *relax* each time you exhale.

C. Scan your body for tension and concentrate on relaxing the muscles that you don't need to continue your activity. For example, if you are sitting at a computer, you can consciously relax the lower part of your body, your abdomen, and much of your head. The muscles in your eyes, back, neck, shoulders, chest, arms, and hands may need to remain somewhat tense for you to look at the monitor and type on the keyboard.

To begin practicing with something like the feeling of your stress reaction, do this exercise after running up a flight of stairs or doing some jumping jacks. When you feel confident, visualize a stressful situation such as a fight with your spouse or an unpleasant encounter with your boss. (Chapter 6 provides ideas and exercises to help you build your visualization skills.) Then practice the three steps of applied relaxation when you encounter a stressful situation in real life. Take a brief moment to collect yourself and remember the three steps, and then put them into effect immediately. No one but you needs to know what you're doing, and you and those around you will all benefit from the calmness with which you approach the crisis at hand.

Be patient with yourself. Applied relaxation is a skill, and you will refine your ability with practice. Note that the chances are good that you won't feel complete relief the first time you try to cut through a deeply stressful situation with applied relaxation. Observe the improvements that you do make. Most people are able to stop anxiety from increasing with relatively little practice. From that point, it's just a few short steps to actually decreasing the anxiety and replacing panic with a feeling of calmness and control.

Special Considerations

If you have progressed methodically from one step of applied relaxation to the next, by now you should have the control you need to bring your body to a state of deep and full relaxation.

As with any other skill, you'll want to practice applied relaxation regularly to keep yourself in top form. Make it a habit to scan your body for tension at least once a day. Focus on ridding your body of that tension using the rapid-relaxation technique. Whatever activity you may be engaged in, you can bring yourself to a calm and deep relaxation.

If there are times when your anxiety doesn't seem to respond or you worry that you've forgotten the skill you once had, remember that setbacks do happen. No treatment can guarantee permanent freedom from anxiety attacks or stress. View setbacks as an opportunity to practice applied relaxation. At other times, enjoy the feeling of deep relaxation that you have achieved. Remind yourself that you can bring yourself there whenever you need to.

You may find it useful to make an audio recording to guide yourself through the exercises described in this chapter. A recording will help you focus on relaxing your body and free you to close your eyes. To make a recording, use the instructions for each step as your script. Speak in a slow, even voice and be sure not to rush through the process.

Another way to learn applied relaxation is to practice it following the instructions on the audio-tape *Applied Relaxation Training* (see Recording).

Further Reading

Öst, L. G. 1987. "Applied Relaxation: Description of a Coping Technique and Review of Controlled Studies." *Behavior Research and Therapy* 25 (5): 397–409.

———. 1988. "Applied Relaxation Vs. Progressive Relaxation in the Treatment of Panic Disorder." *Behavior Research and Therapy* 26 (1): 13–22.

Recording

McKay, M., and P. Fanning. 2008. *Applied Relaxation Training* (Audio CD). Oakland, CA: New Harbinger Publications.

CHAPTER 8

Self-Hypnosis

In this chapter you will learn to:

- Use self-suggestions for deep relaxation and positive change

- Fight stress and stress-related illnesses

- Alleviate specific problems such as insomnia

Background

Hypnosis is a term derived from the Greek word for sleep. In some ways, hypnosis is similar to sleep: there is a narrowing of consciousness accompanied by inertia and passivity. Hypnosis is very relaxing. But unlike sleep, you never completely lose awareness during hypnosis. While hypnotized, you are able to respond to things going on around you. Although hypnosis is usually done with eyes closed to facilitate concentration and imagination, it also can be done with the eyes open.

Hypnosis allows you to experience your thoughts and images as real. While you are hypnotized, you willingly suspend disbelief for the moment, just as you do when you become absorbed in a compelling fantasy or play. For instance, when you watch a violent chase scene in a movie, your mind and body respond in many ways as though you were actually participating in the chase: your muscles tense, your stomach churns, your heart rate increases, and you feel excited or scared. The brain-wave patterns traced on an electroencephalogram (EEG) during hypnosis resemble the patterns that typically occur during the actual activities that the hypnotized person is imagining (participating in a chase, relaxing at the beach, playing a musical instrument, and so on).

You may think that you have never been hypnotized but, in fact, you are no stranger to hypnosis. Often, when you concentrate on something of great interest to you, you enter hypnosis without any formal induction. Daydreaming, for example, is a hypnotic state. Long-distance driving is highly conducive to hypnosis (and commonly results in amnesia for various parts of the trip). You may have entered a form of light hypnosis many times while trying to remember a shopping list, a past sequence of events, or while watching TV and feeling a strong emotion such as fear.

In this chapter you will learn to use self-hypnosis to experience positive thoughts and images of your own choosing for the purpose of relaxing and reducing stress. You can learn self-hypnosis quickly and safely. There are no reported cases of harm resulting from self-hypnosis. Because hypnosis is your experience of your own thoughts and images, it can take place only when your participation is active and voluntary. (This is true even when you are undergoing hypnotic induction by someone else.) You can extend, modify, or shorten any of the hypnosis exercises in this chapter to meet your specific needs.

Symptom-Relief Effectiveness

Self-hypnosis has been clinically effective with symptoms of insomnia, minor chronic pain, headache, nervous tics and tremors, chronic muscular tension, and minor anxiety. It is a well-established treatment for chronic fatigue. You may also consider using self-hypnosis for any subjective experience that could be improved with positive words and images (for example, the rapid heartbeat, cold sweaty palms, and knotted stomach associated with anticipatory anxiety).

Contraindications

Poor candidates for hypnosis include people who are disoriented due to organic brain syndrome or psychosis, people who are severely mentally retarded, and people who are paranoid or hypervigilant.

Time to Master

Significant relaxation effects can be achieved within two days. To become proficient in the skill of self-hypnosis, practice the basic hypnotic induction once a day for a week. Then adapt the basic induction to your personal goals by adding specific hypnotic suggestions. Plan on practicing this modified induction until you no longer need to practice because you will have mastered the skill.

Instructions

The Power of Suggestion

The first step in self-hypnosis is to appreciate the power of suggestion. Here are two simple exercises that can demonstrate the power of suggestion:

Postural Sway

1. Stand up with your eyes closed and imagine holding a suitcase in your right hand.

2. Imagine bigger and bigger suitcases weighing down your right side, pulling you over.

3. After two or three minutes, open your eyes and notice any changes in your posture.

4. Close your eyes again and imagine that the north wind is blowing you, pushing you back on your heels. Feel the gusts. Notice if your weight is shifting in response to your imagination.

Postural Suggestion

1. Stretch both of your arms in front of you at shoulder level. With eyes closed, imagine a weight being tied onto your right arm as it strains to stay up.

2. Imagine a second weight, and then a third. Feel the strain in your arm as it gets heavier and heavier, heavier and heavier.

3. Now imagine that a huge balloon filled with helium has been tied to your left arm and is tugging it up into the air…higher and higher…higher and higher.

4. Open your eyes and notice where your arms are relative to each other.

Most people who try these two exercises notice that their bodies move at least a little in response to these self-suggestions. If you don't notice any movement, practice the exercises a few more times. If you still don't notice even the slightest amount of movement, hypnosis may not be for you.

Personalized Self-Induction

The second step in self-hypnosis is to learn how to write a self-induction script. The following suggestions will provide you with a basic outline for self-induction that you can adapt and change to suit your particular style and purposes.

Position. If possible, sit in a reclining chair or comfortable high-backed chair with support for your arms, hands, neck, and head. Choose a comfortable position with your feet flat on the floor and your legs and arms uncrossed. Loosen your clothing. You may prefer to remove contact lenses or glasses.

Time. Set aside at least thirty minutes to do this exercise without being interrupted.

Key word or phrase. Choose something that is the opposite of your problem and hence the essence of the goal for which you are using hypnosis. For instance, if your problem is anxiety prior to giving a public presentation, your goal and key phrase might be "Calm and clear" or "Relax now." You can repeat this statement slowly at the moment your eyes close and when you are imagining that you are in your special place (see below), so that the key word becomes associated with deep relaxation. A meaningful key phrase may occur to you spontaneously when you experience being in your special place during hypnosis. With enough practice, this key word or phrase will be sufficient to induce hypnosis quickly.

Breathing. After closing your eyes, take several deep breaths. Breathe deeply all the way down into your abdomen and feel the spreading sense of relaxation as you exhale.

Muscle relaxation. You will be relaxing your legs, arms, face, neck, shoulders, chest, and abdomen, in that order. As you relax your legs and arms, the key phrase is "heavier and heavier, more and more deeply relaxed." As you relax your forehead and cheeks, the key phrase is "smooth and relaxed, letting go of tension." As you relax your jaw, the key phrase is "loose and relaxed." Your neck, too, becomes "loose and relaxed." Your shoulders are "relaxed and drooping." You relax your chest, abdomen, and back by first taking a deep breath. As you exhale, use the key phrase "calm and relaxed."

Staircase or path to a special place. You will count each step going down to that peaceful place, and with each step you will become more and more relaxed. Count backward slowly from ten to zero. Each number you count is a step going down. Imagine that saying each number and taking each step helps you to feel more deeply relaxed. You can count backward from ten to zero once, twice, or even three times. Each complete count will deepen your relaxation.

Your special place. Your special place can be any place you feel secure and at peace, for instance, a meadow or beach or your bedroom. When you arrive at your special place, you'll look around and notice the shapes and colors. You'll listen to the sounds and smell the fragrances of your special place. You will also notice the temperature and how your body feels there.

Practice imagining being in your special place before attempting your first self-induction. Make sure that the image is detailed and evocative. If you are at the beach, make sure you can hear the waves crashing and hear the hiss of foam as the waves recede. See and hear the seagulls overhead. Notice the salty sea breeze, the warmth of the sun on your body, and the feel of the sand beneath you. Try to involve all your senses in building the scene: sight, sound, taste, smell, and touch.

Deepening hypnosis. Use the following four key suggestions over and over, in various combinations, until you feel a deep sense of calm and letting go.

1. *Drifting deeper and deeper, deeper and deeper*

2. *Feeling more and more drowsy, peaceful, and calm*

3. *Drifting and drowsy, drowsy and drifting*

4. *Drifting down, down, down into total relaxation*

Posthypnotic suggestion. Once you've spent time relaxing in your special place, you may wish to give yourself posthypnotic suggestions. Later in this chapter, the sections Hypnotic Suggestions and Practice Writing Hypnotic Suggestions provide tips on how to craft posthypnotic suggestions.

Coming out of hypnosis. When it's time to end your trance, you can count back up from one to ten. In between numbers, tell yourself that you are becoming "more and more alert, refreshed, and wide awake." As you reach number nine, tell yourself that your eyes are opening. As you say the number ten, tell yourself that you are totally alert and wide awake.

Here is a summary of the key rules for a successful self-induction:

1. Allow at least twenty minutes to enter and deepen the hypnotic state.

2. Don't worry about success or how you are doing. Hypnosis will become easier with practice.

3. Always allow time to relax your muscles and take deep breaths.

4. Use compelling instructions ("I am feeling more and more heaviness in my arms").

5. Use adjectives such as "drowsy," "peaceful," or "comfortable" during self-induction.

6. Repeat everything until the suggestion begins to take hold.

7. Use creative imagery. For example, to induce heaviness, imagine your legs as lead pipes. For lightness, imagine helium-filled balloons pulling up your arm or imagine floating on a cloud.

Basic Self-Induction Script

The third step to self-hypnosis is to record the basic script below and play it back for your initial inductions. When you read the induction aloud, speak in a monotone. Keep the tempo slow and monotonous. Pronounce one word after another with an even beat. Pause between each sentence. Speaking slowly, with little inflection, will help your mind drift and increase your relaxation and suggestibility. After some experience with this induction, you will be ready to write your own personalized self-induction.

> *Sit in a comfortable position with your arms and legs uncrossed. Let your eyes focus gently on a point in front of you…take a deep, relaxing breath all the way down into your abdomen.… Take another slow, deep, relaxing breath…and another.… Even though your eyes are getting tired, keep them open a little longer and take another deep breath…and another.… Your eyes become heavier and heavier…let them close, as you say to yourself* [Insert your key word or phrase here].

Now you can begin to relax the muscles in your body. Let your legs begin to relax…let your legs begin to feel heavy…heavier and heavier as they relax. Your legs are heavier and heavier as they let go of the last bit of muscular tension.… Your legs are becoming more and more heavy and relaxed, heavy and relaxed.… Your arms, too, are becoming more and more heavy… heavier and heavier as they let go of the last bit of muscular tension. You can feel gravity pulling them down.… You feel your arms growing heavier and heavier, more and more deeply relaxed. Your arms are letting go…letting go…letting go of tension as they become heavier and heavier… more and more deeply relaxed. Your arms and legs feel heavy, heavy, and relaxed.… Your arms and legs feel totally relaxed as they let go of the last bit of muscular tension…more and more heavy and relaxed.…

And your face, too, begins to relax. Your forehead is becoming smooth and relaxed. Your forehead is letting go of tension as it becomes more and more smooth and relaxed.… And your cheeks too are becoming relaxed, smooth and relaxed. Your cheeks are relaxed and letting go of tension…your forehead and cheeks are totally relaxed…smooth and relaxed .… And your jaw can now begin to relax…feeling more and more loose and relaxed. As your jaw becomes more and more deeply relaxed, feel the muscles letting go…and your lips beginning to part…and your jaw becoming more and more loose and relaxed.

Now your neck and shoulders can begin to relax. Your neck is loose and relaxed…your shoulders are relaxed and drooping.… Feel your neck and shoulders becoming more and more deeply relaxed…so loose and relaxed.… Now, take another deep breath, and as you exhale let the relaxation spread into your chest and stomach and back.… Take another deep breath and, as you exhale, feel yourself becoming calm and relaxed…calm and relaxed. Take another deep breath…and as you exhale, feel your chest and stomach and back become calm and relaxed… calm and relaxed. Feel yourself drifting deeper and deeper…deeper and deeper…becoming more and more drowsy, peaceful, and calm. Drifting and drowsy…drowsy and drifting…drifting down, down, down into total relaxation…drifting deeper and deeper…deeper and deeper.

Now it's time to go to your special place…a place of safety and peace. You can go down the stairway to your special place or down a path, and with each step you can count backward from ten to zero…and with each step become more and more deeply relaxed. In ten steps you will be there…feeling peaceful and safe as you move toward your special place. Now you grow more and more relaxed with each step. Ten…nine…eight…seven…six…five…four…three…two… one…zero.

[If you want to repeat this countdown two or even three times to deepen hypnosis, that's perfectly fine.]

Now see the shapes and colors of your special place…hear the sounds…feel the sensations of your special place…smell the smells of your special place. See it…feel it…hear it…smell it.… You can feel safe and calm in your special place, safe and calm.…

Feel yourself drifting deeper and deeper, deeper and deeper…more and more drowsy, peaceful, and calm. You feel drowsy and drifting, drifting and drowsy…drifting down, down, down into total relaxation. You are so relaxed, peaceful, and calm.

[Pause and spend time relaxing in your special place.]

Now you know that you can...

[Leave a blank space on the tape here for any posthypnotic suggestion that you wish to use. Give yourself time to repeat the suggestion at least three times.]

Now, when you are ready, it is time to come back up...to come all the way back, feeling alert, refreshed, and wide awake. Starting to come up now: one...two...three...four...more and more alert and aware...five...six...seven...more and more alert and awake...eight...nine... beginning to open your eyes...and ten...completely alert, refreshed, and wide awake. Alert, refreshed, and wide awake.

Abbreviated Inductions

An optional fourth step to self-hypnosis is to learn to do *abbreviated inductions*. These are shorthand techniques that can produce hypnosis in thirty seconds to two minutes. Here are some examples.

Pendulum drop. To make a pendulum, tie an object like a paper clip, pen, or ring to the end of a heavy thread ten inches long. Hold the thread in your dominant hand and let the pendulum dangle above the floor. Ask your subconscious for permission to go into hypnosis for two minutes. If the answer is yes, your eyes will want to close. As your eyes close, picture a candle flame. Take several deep breaths and allow yourself to slip into a deeper and deeper relaxation. Tell yourself that when you have entered hypnosis, your hand will relax and drop the pendulum. Count down slowly from ten to zero.

Yes repetition. Think the thought *yes* over and over as you focus on an imagined candle flame. Go down the stairs or down a path to your special place while you continue to think *yes*.

Eye fixation. Fix your eyes on a point slightly above your normal line of vision. Let your peripheral vision narrow and your eyes lose focus. Allow your eyes to close, accompanied by a feeling of drowsiness. To increase the drowsiness, roll your eyes up to the top of your head two or three times.

Key word or phrase. Breathe deeply and slowly, and repeat the key word or phrase that you used in your self-induction script. As you say the word or phrase, close your eyes and enter hypnosis.

These abbreviated methods are useful after you have become relatively proficient at self-hypnosis. Always remember to end an induction by suggesting that you will awaken refreshed and feeling fine.

Five-finger exercise. The next exercise has been used very effectively for relaxation. Memorize the following steps. After you have gone through them, you can use the feeling of calmness that follows to enter hypnosis.

1. Touch your thumb to your index finger. As you do that, go back to a time when your body felt healthy fatigue, such as just after swimming, playing tennis, jogging, or some other exhilarating physical activity.

2. Touch your thumb to your middle finger. As you do that, go back to a time when you had a loving experience. You may choose to remember a moment of sexual fulfillment, a warm embrace, or an intimate conversation.

3. Touch your thumb to your ring finger. As you do that, recall the nicest compliment you have ever received. Try to really accept it now. By accepting it, you are showing your high regard for the person who said it. You are really paying that person a compliment in return.

4. Touch your thumb to your little finger. As you do that, go back to the most beautiful place you have ever been. Dwell there for a while.

The five-finger exercise takes less than ten minutes, but it pays off with increased vitality, inner peace, and self-esteem. It can be done any time you feel tension.

Hypnotic Suggestions

A fifth useful step to self-hypnosis is to learn how to give yourself positive suggestions for change. For best results, say these suggestions to yourself when you are in a relaxed and receptive frame of mind, such as when you are in your special place during the basic self-induction. Or you may find that you prefer to intersperse suggestions throughout an induction.

Remember that autosuggestions are thoughts and images that influence your subjective experience. Here's a list of rules to keep in mind when you are creating suggestions for yourself:

Autosuggestions are most effective when they are:

1. *Direct.* Tell yourself, "I will be calm, confident, and in control."

2. *Positive.* Avoid negative wording, such as "I won't feel tired tonight."

3. *Permissive.* Try saying "I *can* feel relaxed and refreshed tonight" instead of "I *will* feel relaxed and refreshed." However, some people do respond better to commands. You can experiment with both to find out which approach works best for you.

4. *About the immediate future, not the present.* "Soon the drowsiness is going to come upon me."

5. *Repeated at least three times.*

6. *Represented with a visual image.* If you are trying to overcome a feeling of exhaustion, imagine yourself bouncing along with springs on your feet and see yourself as looking athletic and happy.

7. *Reinforced with an emotion or a sensation.* If you want to give up smoking cigarettes, imagine how bad the first one tasted or think of the unpleasant burning in your lungs. If you are attempting to improve your confidence for a first date, imagine the feeling of closeness and belonging that you are hoping to find.

8. *Not associated with the word "try."* That's because "try" implies doubt and the possibility of failure.

9. *Exaggerated at first when working toward the control of unpleasant emotions or painful physical symptoms.* Start out by suggesting that the negative emotion or symptom is growing more intense. You might say, "My anger is getting bigger. I can feel the blood pushing at my veins. I'm getting hot. My muscles are tensing." Bring the feeling up to a peak and then tell yourself that the emotion or symptom is diminishing. "My anger is subsiding. My heart is slowing and beating normally. My flush is receding. My muscles are loosening and beginning to relax." When an unpleasant emotion or symptom reaches its peak, it can only get better. Suggestion can speed that process of recovery. When you can turn your emotions and symptoms on and off during hypnosis, you will have gained enormous control over your life.

10. *Written out in advance.* After you've written it out, distill it into a catchword or phrase you can easily remember when you are in the hypnotic state.

Practice Writing Hypnotic Suggestions

Once hypnotized and relaxed, your subconscious mind is more open to believing whatever you tell it. Many of the symptoms that bother you, as well as your habitual tension responses to stress, were learned through suggestion. They can be unlearned through suggestion. For example, if you watched your father get angry every time he was forced to wait, and if on the first occasion when you delayed him, he became angry with you, you may have learned by suggestion to respond exactly the same way. You can use hypnosis to learn new methods of coping with delay. Suggestions such as "Waiting is a chance to relax" and "I can let go of rushing" may undo the old habit.

In order to get the flavor of how suggestions can be written, write down hypnotic suggestions that you could use for the following problems:

1. Fear of coming into a dark house at night

2. Chronic fatigue

3. Obsessive and fearful thoughts about death

4. Fear of illness

5. Minor chronic head or back pain

6. Chronic anger and/or guilt

7. Self-criticism and worry about making mistakes

8. Low self-esteem

9. Lack of motivation

10. Feelings of insecurity and self-consciousness in the presence of other people

11. Anxiety about an upcoming evaluation or test

12. Improving performance

13. Pain or muscle tension

14. Disease and injury

Now that you have written your own suggestions, examine these possible scripts for each of the fourteen problems.

1. Fear of coming into a dark house at night

    I can come in tonight feeling relaxed and glad to be home, safe, and secure.

2. Chronic fatigue

    I can awaken refreshed and rested. I can enjoy the evening ahead. I can pace myself today so that I will accomplish my priorities. Whenever I feel my energy flagging, I can do the five-finger exercise or another relaxation technique and then return to my daily activities relaxed and revitalized.

3. Obsessive and fearful thoughts about death

    I am full of life now. I will enjoy today. Very soon I can let go of these thoughts. (Visualize a blackboard and see the date written there.)

4. Fear of illness

    My body is feeling healthy and strong more and more. Each time I relax, my body becomes stronger. (Visualize yourself as healthy, strong, and relaxed while doing a favorite activity.)

5. Minor chronic head or back pain

    Soon my head will be cool and relaxed. (Imagine cool images.) *Gradually I will feel the muscles in my neck and back loosen.* (Imagine smooth, flowing, loosening images.) *In an hour, they will be completely relaxed. Whenever these symptoms come back, I will simply turn my ring a quarter turn to the right and the pain will relax away.*

6. Chronic anger and/or guilt

    I can turn off anger and guilt because I am the one who turns it on. (Practice turning up and turning down the unwanted emotion.) *I will relax my body and breathe deeply.*

7. Self-criticism and worry about making mistakes

When I catch myself being self-critical or worried, I can take a deep breath and let go. I can breathe out negative tension and breathe in positive energy. (Practice five-finger exercise.)

8. Low self-esteem

Each day I will feel more capable and self-assured. I can do it. I am doing the best I can with my prevailing level of awareness. I can feel myself becoming happier and more successful every day. I can be kind to myself. I am liking myself more and more. I am an intelligent, creative, and talented person.

9. Lack of motivation

I can feel confident that I will achieve my goals. I have the power within myself to change. I can see myself solving my problems and getting beyond them. The decisions I make are the right ones for now. I can put aside distractions and focus my attention on one goal. As I get into my project, I will get more and more interested in it. As I work toward my goal, step by step, new energy and enthusiasm will emerge. When I finish this, I will feel great! When I achieve my goal, I will reward myself. I deserve success.

10. Feelings of insecurity and self-consciousness in the presence of other people

The next time I see Ben, I can feel secure in myself. I can respond to Ben in a firm and assertive manner. I can feel relaxed and at ease because I am perfectly all right. I can relax and enjoy the thought that there are people in my life who see me as a good friend, valuable coworker, and loving family member. Whenever I lace my fingers together, I will feel confidence flowing throughout my entire body.

11. Anxiety about an upcoming evaluation or test

I can concentrate on my studies, remembering everything I need to know for the test. When I feel nervous, I will take a deep breath and relax. My mind is becoming more and more calm and sharp. When I successfully complete this test, I will reward myself with _____. I can imagine myself getting an A.

12. Improving performance

I can be calm and in control in response to stressful situations. (Imagine yourself maintaining your cool and concentration in the face of specific pressures and fears.) *I can imagine myself playing a perfect game from start to finish.* (Reflect on every perfect move and strategy.) *I will achieve my goal.* (Be specific about your objectives and visualize them in detail.)

13. Pain or muscle tension

I can see my back pain as a sword of dry ice burning and stabbing me. Now I see the sun shining, warming my back. The ice sword is gradually melting away into a puddle in the warmth of the sun, and my pain is beginning to subside. My tension is starting to flow; as it flows, its color changes into a warm orange fluid moving slowly through my body toward my right shoulder, down my right arm, and into my clenched fist. When I am ready, I can let go of it. I can just scoop my pain up and throw it away. (Imagine a symbol that best represents your pain or tension. Have it interact with another symbol that eliminates the first symbol or transforms it into something more tolerable or makes it disappear.)

14. Disease and injury

I can imagine a healing white light at the top of my head. I can see and feel it surrounding my entire body. I can feel it begin to move within my body, cleansing and healing as it slowly spreads throughout my entire body. I can imagine myself healthy, strong, and energetic while doing what I want to do.

Self-Hypnotic Induction for a Specific Problem

Another optional step is to consider how self-hypnosis might fit into an overall plan to solve a specific problem in your life. The specific problem addressed here is sleep disturbance. This section is adapted from Josie Hadley and Carol Staudacher's *Hypnosis for Change* (1996).

Before you are ready to begin self-hypnosis for a specific problem, there are a few issues you need to address. They are as follows:

Define your problem and your goal. Do you have difficulty falling asleep or staying asleep, or do you wake up too early? Is your sleep restless? Do you have great difficulty waking up in the morning? Once you have clearly labeled your problem, you can easily define your goal in the form of a positive autosuggestion. For example, "I can fall asleep quickly and easily." "I will wake up refreshed and alert at the appropriate time." Or "Soon I will be able to sleep deeply and continuously throughout the night."

Identify and eliminate any possible external factors that may be contributing to your problem. Ask yourself what might be interfering with getting a good night's sleep. Is your bedroom a comfortable place that invites sleep, or is it filled with clutter, noise, and light? Do you spend half the night coping with a restless bed partner and staring at a glowing clock face that keeps reminding you of how much sleep you are losing? Are you consuming too many stimulants during the day? You need to address these problems before using self-hypnosis for better sleep, because you cannot expect self-hypnosis to solve these problems for you.

Notice what you are telling yourself that may be contributing to your problem. For example, people who have difficulty with sleep often focus on time. They say things to themselves like, *If I don't get to sleep by midnight, I know I won't be able to sleep at all.* If you tend to worry, your mind can go wild when you turn off the light. *I really blew it today. Wait until my boss finds out!* Or *I know I didn't study enough for the test tomorrow.* Do you use the quiet hours of the night to solve problems?

Until this question is answered, we can't go on! Or I'll tell her I didn't mean what I said, and then she'll say…

If part of your problem has to do with what you are telling yourself, you can use the chapters "Refuting Irrational Ideas," "Relieving Worry and Anxiety," and "Anger Inoculation" to help you identify and change the way you think. If you are being kept awake by your thoughts, here are some suggestions to calm your mind before you fall asleep.

- If you are a clock-watcher, turn the clock to the wall, direct your thoughts away from time, and tell yourself, "As I rest, my mind will become calm and my body will relax."

- If you tend to dwell on the negative or on things that you cannot control, think about the positive things you did during the day.

- If you are a nighttime problem solver, write your to-do list *before* you go to bed and then make an agreement with yourself to put aside your problems until tomorrow when you are at your sharpest and to save the night for restorative sleep.

When you create your own sleep induction, be sure to write in positive suggestions that incorporate these ideas to reinforce your new desired behavior.

Record an induction tailored to your particular problem. Begin by recording the basic induction up through the section about your special place, and then add your special suggestions. For sleep disturbance, you might add the following script to the basic induction.

Now just linger in your special place. There's no place to go, nothing to do. Just rest, just let yourself drift and float, drift and float into a sound and restful sleep. And as you drift deeper and deeper, imagine the positive things that you can think and do to allow yourself a sound and restful sleep. Your new positive thoughts are true. You have released negative thoughts and feelings. You have released stress and tension from your mind and body. Each new positive statement becomes stronger and stronger as you continue to drift deeper and deeper into relaxation. Just let yourself drift deeper and deeper into sleep. Just let those positive statements float in your mind as you drift into a sound and restful sleep.

Now become aware of how comfortable you feel, so relaxed, your head and shoulders are in just the right position, your back is supported, and you are becoming less aware of all the normal sounds of your surroundings. As you drift deeper and deeper, you may experience a negative thought or worry that is trying to surface in your mind and disrupt your slumber and your rest. Simply take that thought and sweep it up as you would sweep up crumbs from the floor and place that thought or worry into a box. The box has a nice tight lid. Put the lid on the box and place the box on the top shelf of your closet. You can go back to that box at another time, a time that is more appropriate, a time that will not interfere with your sleep. As other unwanted thoughts appear, sweep them up and place them in the box, put the lid on the box, and place it on the top shelf of your closet to let them go. Let them go and continue to drift deeper and deeper into sleep.

Shift your thoughts back to your positive thoughts and positive statements. Just let these thoughts flow through your mind, thoughts such as, "I am a worthwhile person." (Pause.) "I have accomplished many good things." (Pause.) "I have reached positive goals." (Pause.) Just let your positive ideas flow through your mind. Let them flow and drift, becoming stronger and stronger as you drift deeper and deeper into sleep.

You may begin to see them slowly fade, slowly fade, as you become even more relaxed, sleepier, more drowsy, more relaxed. Just imagine yourself in your peaceful and special place, smiling, feeling so good, so comfortable, so relaxed. (Pause.) From your special place you can easily drift into a sound and restful sleep, a sound and restful sleep, undisturbed in a sound and restful sleep. You sleep through the night in a sound and restful sleep. If you should awaken, you simply imagine your special place once again and drift easily back into a sound and restful sleep, a sound and restful sleep. Your breathing becomes so relaxed, your thoughts wind down, wind down, wind down, and relax. You drift and float into a sound and restful sleep, undisturbed throughout the night. You will awaken at your designated time feeling rested and refreshed.

Now there's nothing to do, nothing to think about, nothing to do but enjoy your special place, your special place that is so peaceful for you, so relaxing. Just imagine how it feels to relax in your special place. You may become aware of how clean and fresh your special place smells, or you may become aware of the different sounds of your special place, of the birds singing in the background or the water cascading over river rocks in a stream. Or you may become aware of how warm the sun feels as you lounge in a hammock or how cool the breeze feels from the ocean air. Or you may experience something else that is unique and wonderful in your special place. Just experience it, drift and float, all thought just fading, drifting into a sound and restful sleep. Just drift into a comfortable, cozy, restful sleep, your body feeling heavy and relaxed as you sink into your bed, so relaxed, just drifting into sleep…sleep…sleep…sleep…sleep…sleep….

Special Considerations

Do not practice a hypnotic induction in a car or in any other situation where your safety requires you to be fully alert and able to respond quickly. After an induction, always make sure that you are completely awake and alert before reentering such situations.

Some people, especially those who are sleep-deprived, fall asleep during self-hypnosis. If sleep is not your goal and you have this problem, you may want to shorten the induction so that you are awake to hear the suggestions specifically geared to your goals. Keep in mind that many people who think they are asleep during hypnosis are still able to hear and benefit from positive suggestions. If you are prone to falling asleep, practice it sitting up and use a timer to wake yourself up rather than worry about being late for your next activity.

You may find that as the symptom you are concerned about fades, you lose your motivation to continue practicing self-hypnosis. This is a typical experience and nothing to worry about. If your symptom returns at a later time, you can use self-hypnosis again.

You can use your key phrase when you experience your symptom or any time you feel tense or uncomfortable in a stressful situation. Although you are unlikely to feel as relaxed as you do after a full self-hypnotic induction, you will still experience some measure of relief. In this way, your key phrase can also serve as a reminder that you do have a choice about how you respond to stress.

Whether you are using self-hypnosis to relax or to accomplish some other goal, you are likely to be pleasantly surprised by the power of positive suggestion.

Further Reading

Alman, B. M., and P. Lambrou. 1992. *Self-Hypnosis: The Complete Manual for Health and Self-Change.* 2nd ed. New York: Brunner-Mazel.

Hadley, J., and C. Staudacher. 1996. *Hypnosis for Change: A Manual of Proven Techniques.* 3rd ed. Oakland, CA: New Harbinger Publications.

Haley, J. 1993. *Uncommon Therapy: The Psychiatric Techniques of Milton Erickson.* Reissue ed. New York: W. W. Norton & Company.

Hunter, C. R. 1998. *Master the Power of Self-Hypnosis.* New York: Sterling Publications.

MacKanzie, R. 2005. *Self-Change Hypnosis.* Victoria, BC: Trafford Publishing.

Rosen, S. 1991. *My Voice Will Go with You.* Reprint ed. New York: W. W. Norton & Company.

Soskis, D. A. 1986. *Self-Hypnosis: An Introductory Guide for Clinicians.* New York: W. W. Norton & Company.

CHAPTER 9

Autogenics

In this chapter you will learn to:

- Respond quickly to verbal commands to relax

- Return your body to a balanced, normal state

- Calm your mind

- Resolve specific physical problems

Background

Autogenic training (AT) has its origins in research on hypnosis conducted by the famous brain physiologist Oskar Vogt at the Berlin Institute during the last decade of the nineteenth century. Vogt taught some of his experienced hypnotic subjects to put themselves into a trance that had the effect of reducing their fatigue, tension, and painful symptoms like headaches. It also seemed to help the subjects deal more effectively with their everyday lives. They usually reported that when their fatigue and tension lifted, they felt warm and heavy.

Johannes H. Schultz, a Berlin psychiatrist, became interested in Vogt's work. He found that his subjects could create a state very much like a hypnotic trance just by thinking of heaviness and warmth in their extremities. Essentially, all they had to do was relax, be undisturbed, sit in a comfortable position, and concentrate passively on verbal formulas that suggested they feel warmth and heaviness in their limbs. Schultz combined some of Vogt's autosuggestions with some yoga techniques (Schultz and Luthe 1969).

Schultz's verbal formulas fall into four main categories of exercises:

1. Verbal formulas to normalize the body

2. Verbal formulas to calm the mind

3. Autogenic modification exercises designed to address specific problems

4. Meditative exercises to develop mental concentration and creativity

This introductory chapter will teach you to use verbal formulas to relax your body, calm your mind, and help you resolve specific problems.

The verbal formulas to normalize the body are aimed at reversing the fight-or-flight response state, or high-alarm state, that occurs when anyone experiences physical or emotional stress. These formulas fall under six standard themes.

1. The first standard theme is *heaviness*, which promotes relaxation of the voluntary muscles used to move your arms and legs. There are seven verbal formulas that suggest the theme of heaviness (see set 1 under Autogenic Verbal Formulas for Normalizing the Body).

2. The second standard theme is *warmth*, which brings about peripheral *vasodilatation*, the relaxing and widening of the blood vessels, in the hands and feet so that blood flows to them, creating sensations of warmth and heaviness. As you say the verbal formula "My right hand is warm," the smooth muscles that control the diameter of the blood vessels in your hand relax so that more warming blood flows into your hand. This helps reverse the pooling of blood in the trunk and head characteristic of the fight-or-flight reaction to stress.

3. The third standard theme focuses on *normalizing cardiac activity*. The verbal formula is simply "My heartbeat is calm and regular."

4. The fourth standard theme *regulates the respiratory system*. The verbal formula is, "It breathes me."

5. The fifth standard theme *relaxes and warms the abdominal region*. The formula to say is "My solar plexus is warm."

6. The last standard theme *reduces the flow of blood to the head* while you say, "My forehead is cool."

The verbal formulas to calm the mind are used in conjunction with these six themes and serve to intensify the effect of the themes.

Symptom-Relief Effectiveness

Autogenic training has been found to be effective in the treatment of muscle tension and various disorders of the respiratory tract (hyperventilation and bronchial asthma), the gastrointestinal tract (constipation, diarrhea, gastritis, ulcers, and spasms), the circulatory system (racing heart, irregular heartbeat, high blood pressure, cold extremities, and headaches), and the endocrine system (thyroid problems). AT is also useful in reducing general anxiety, irritability, and fatigue. It can be employed to modify your reaction to pain, increase your resistance to stress, and reduce or eliminate sleeping disorders.

Contraindications

Autogenic training is not recommended for children under the age of five, people who lack motivation, or those with severe mental or emotional disorders. Prior to beginning AT, it is essential that you have a physical exam and discussion with your medical doctor about what physiological effects AT will likely have on you. Those with serious diseases such as diabetes, hypoglycemic conditions, or heart conditions should be under the supervision of a medical doctor while in AT. Some people experience an increase in blood pressure and a few have a sharp drop in blood pressure when they do these exercises. If you have high or low blood pressure, you should check with your medical doctor to be sure that AT is regularizing it. If you feel very anxious or restless during or after AT exercises or experience recurring disquieting side effects, you should continue AT only under the supervision of a professional AT instructor.

Time to Master

In the past, autogenic training specialists recommended moving at a slow but sure and steady pace, taking many months to master all six themes. We've found this timetable unrealistic for people who want and typically get some positive results in the very first session of AT. Others require a week or two of regular practice to experience relaxation. Plan on practicing your autogenic formulas at least twice a day for twenty minutes. If you find this is too long for you, shorten the length of the session and add more sessions each day.

By the end of one month of regular practice, you should be able to relax quickly using all six themes. At that time, you may choose to use all six themes in one twenty-minute relaxation exercise or perhaps only a few themes that rapidly bring about deep relaxation for you. For instance, the formulas "My arms and legs are heavy and warm," "My heartbeat is calm and regular," and "It breathes me" may be sufficient to induce immediate relaxation. You should experiment to find what works best for you.

Instructions

How to Facilitate Your Relaxation When Doing AT

- Keep external stimuli to a minimum.

- Choose a quiet room where you won't be disturbed.

- Keep the room temperature at a moderately warm, comfortable level.

- Turn the lights down low.

- Wear loose clothing.

- Choose one of the following three basic AT postures: (1) Sit in an armchair in which your head, back, and extremities are supported and you are as comfortable as possible. (2) Sit on a stool, slightly stooped over, with your arms resting on your thighs, your neck relaxed, and your hands draped between your knees. (3) Lie down on your back with your head supported and your legs about eight inches apart, your toes pointed slightly outward, and your arms resting comfortably at your sides but not touching your body.

- Scan your body to be sure that the position you chose is tension-free. In particular, look for overextension of your limbs such as unsupported arms, head, or legs, tightening of the limbs at the joints, or a crooked spine. If any of these overextensions exist, continue moving and supporting your body until you are well supported and comfortable, with no overextensions.

- Close your eyes or pick a point in front of you to softly focus on.

- Take a few slow, deep, and relaxing breaths before you begin to repeat your autogenic formulas.

How to Practice the Six Basic Autogenic Themes to Normalize Your Body

There are two ways to learn the six basic autogenic themes. The first option is to make a recording of the verbal formulas and listen to it twice a day. Or, you can memorize and practice one set of verbal formulas at a time until you include all of the themes in your practice. Slowly repeat each formula over and over to yourself, keeping up a steady silent verbal stream.

As a general rule of thumb, repeat each formula four times, saying it slowly (taking about five seconds) and then pausing for about three seconds. Using the first three verbal formulas of the first set as an example, you would say to yourself, "My right arm is heavy… My right arm is heavy… My right arm is heavy… My right arm is heavy." This should take you about half a minute. Then you would say to yourself, "My left arm is heavy… My left arm is heavy… My left arm is heavy… My left arm is heavy…" Then, "Both of my arms are heavy… Both of my arms are heavy… Both of my arms are heavy… Both of my arms are heavy…" The entire set should take you less than four minutes. If you are focusing on memorizing one set at a time, you can repeat the set up to twenty minutes in one practice session or create many mini-practice sessions of one or a few sets throughout the day. If you are recording the verbal formulas, be sure to leave about half a minute between each formula for silent repetition.

As you silently repeat a verbal formula, passively concentrate on the part of the body it refers to. In other words, just notice what happens without harboring any expectations or judgments. Passive concentration does not mean spacing out or going to sleep. You remain alert to your experience without analyzing it. This casual attitude is contrasted with active concentration, which occurs when you fix your attention on certain aspects of your experience and have an interest and goal-directed investment in it. *Active concentration* is essential for such tasks as preparing a new recipe or fixing a car. *Passive concentration* is required for relaxation.

At first, you will not be able to maintain perfect passive concentration. Your mind will wander. That's natural. When you find this happening, just return to the formula as soon as possible. In addition, you may experience some initial symptoms known as *autogenic discharges*, which are normal but distracting, such as a change in your weight or temperature, tingling, "electrical currents," involuntary movements, stiffness, some pain, anxiety, a desire to cry, irritability, headaches, nausea, or illusions. At times, you may experience fascinating insights or feelings of bliss. Whether you have pleasant or unpleasant experiences, just note them and return to your AT formulas. Remember that these experiences are transitory, they are not the purpose of AT, and they will pass as you continue to practice.

When you are ready to stop an AT session, say to yourself, "When I open my eyes, I will feel refreshed and alert." Then open your eyes and breathe a few deep breaths as you stretch and flex your arms. Be sure that you are not still in a trancelike state when you return to your regular activities.

Read the helpful hints and cautionary notes in the Special Considerations section at the end of this chapter before you begin to practice AT. The following set of autogenic verbal formulas is available at http://www.newharbinger.com/43348.

Autogenic Verbal Formulas for Normalizing the Body

Set 1

My right arm is heavy.

My left arm is heavy.

Both of my arms are heavy.

My right leg is heavy.

My left leg is heavy.

Both of my legs are heavy.

My arms and legs are heavy.

Set 2

My right arm is warm.

My left arm is warm.

Both of my arms are warm.

My right leg is warm.

Both of my legs are warm.

My arms and legs are warm.

Set 3

My right arm is heavy and warm.

Both of my arms are heavy and warm.

Both of my legs are heavy and warm.

My arms and legs are heavy and warm.

It breathes me.

My heartbeat is calm and regular.

Set 4

My right arm is heavy and warm.

My arms and legs are heavy and warm.

It breathes me.

My heartbeat is calm and regular.

My solar plexus is warm.

Set 5

My right arm is heavy and warm.

My arms and legs are heavy and warm.

It breathes me.

My heartbeat is calm and regular.

My solar plexus is warm.

My arms and legs are warm.

My forehead is cool.

Autogenic Formulas for Calming the Mind

The following formulas focus on mental rather than physical functions. They are intended to reinforce the effects of the autogenic verbal formulas for the six standard themes previously mentioned. Here is a list of examples:

I am calm and relaxed.

I feel quite quiet.

My whole body feels quiet, heavy, comfortable, and relaxed.

My mind is quiet.

I withdraw my thoughts from the surroundings and I feel serene and still.

My thoughts are turned inward and I am at ease.

Deep within my mind, I can visualize and experience myself as relaxed and comfortable and still.

I feel an inward quietness.

You may add one or more of these phrases for calming the mind at the end of each set of autogenic verbal formulas. But for the best results, intersperse them throughout each set. For example, the first set could be rewritten as follows:

My right arm is heavy.

I am calm and relaxed.

My left arm is heavy.

I am calm and relaxed.

Both of my arms are heavy.

I am calm and relaxed.

My right leg is heavy.

I am calm and relaxed.

My left leg is heavy.

I am calm and relaxed.

Both of my legs are heavy.

I am calm and relaxed.

Autogenic Modification Exercises

You can practice autogenic modification by making up what Schultz called "organ-specific formulae" to deal with specific problems after you have mastered the six basic autogenic themes. For example, you can develop an *indirect formula,* such as "My feet are warm" or "My shoulders are warm," each time you feel an embarrassing blush coming on. This allows you to passively attend to something other than the problem of blushing. At the same time, you move some of the blood from your head that would contribute to the blushing toward your feet. You might also use a *direct formula,* such as "My forehead is cool."

When you experience persistent muscle pain or tension in a specific part of your body, use the autogenic verbal formulas to become generally relaxed. Then passively concentrate on the persistently tense or painful area and project the sensation of comfortably warm relaxation into that area. Repeat to yourself, "My [name of tense or painful area] is warm and comfortably relaxed."

If you have a headache, concentrate on the area that tends to tighten up most at the beginning of a headache. For instance, if it is your shoulders or neck or back of the head, passively concentrate on that area and project the sensation of warm relaxation into it, repeating to yourself, "My [name of tense area] is warm and comfortably relaxed." Occasionally, intersperse the formula with "My forehead feels comfortably cool." Never make the suggestion "My forehead feels warm," because that would stimulate vasodilatation in the area, which could result in pain.

When you are troubled by a cough, you may want to use the verbal formula "My throat is cool, my chest is warm." To cope with asthma, use the same formula and add, "It breathes me, it breathes me calm and regular."

When you are in a very relaxed state toward the end of an AT session, you are highly suggestible. This is a good time to use what Schultz called "intentional formulae." In other words, you tell yourself to stop doing things that have been causing you difficulties. For example, if you want to stop smoking, say something over and over again, such as, "Smoking is a dirty habit, and I can do without it." If you want to eat less, say, "I have control over what I eat. I can eat less and be more attractive." These special intentional formulas should be believable, persuasive, and brief.

Special Considerations

1. When practicing the six basic autogenic themes, start with your dominant arm: if you write with your left hand, begin with your left arm. Repeat "My left arm is heavy" four times and then go on to the next phrase, "My right arm is heavy," and repeat it four times, and so on.

2. If you have trouble experiencing the physical sensations suggested by the verbal formulas, try imagery. Contemplate being in a nice warm shower or bath or having your hand submerged in a comfortably warm pan of water. Feel yourself sitting in the warm sun or holding a nice warm mug of your favorite hot drink in your hand. Think about blood flowing gently through the fingertips of your hands and through your toes. Imagine lying under a

comfortably heavy warm blanket or lying under the warm, heavy sand at the beach. Recall a cool breeze or washcloth on your forehead.

3. Note that perhaps 10 percent of all people experimenting with AT never experience the basic sensations of heaviness or warmth. This doesn't matter. The formulas describing warmth and heaviness are used only to bring about a functional change in the body, which you may or may not feel. Just focus on doing the formulas correctly, and within two weeks of regular practice, you should experience feelings of relaxation.

4. Some people experience a paradoxical response when they first practice the autogenic verbal formulas. For example, they feel light as they repeat the verbal formulas for heaviness, or they feel cool as they say the formulas for warmth. This is an indication that the body is responding to the formulas and will in time relax.

5. If you feel stuck or are experiencing unpleasant side effects while practicing one of the themes, move on to the next one and come back to the formula that is difficult for you at the end of your training period.

6. If you have trouble becoming aware of your heartbeat, lie on your back with your right hand resting over your heart. If you experience any discomfort or distress while becoming aware of your heartbeat, move on to another theme and come back to this one at the end of your training session, or skip it.

7. Skip the verbal formula "My solar plexus is warm" if you have ulcers, diabetes, or any condition involving bleeding from abdominal organs. If you notice dizziness or light-headedness when you practice the verbal formula "My forehead is cool," practice it lying down.

Further Reading

Goleman, D., and J. Gurin, eds. 1993. *Mind Body Medicine: How to Use Your Mind for Better Health*. Yonkers, NY: Consumer Reports Books.

Kermani, K. 1996. *Autogenic Training: The Effective Holistic Way to Better Health*. Reissue ed. London: Souvenir Press.

Linden, W. 1990. *Autogenics: A Clinical Guide*. New York: Guilford Press.

Pelletier, K. R. 1977. *Mind As Healer, Mind As Slayer*. New York: Delta.

Peurifory, R. Z. 2005. *Anxiety, Phobias, and Panic: Taking Charge and Conquering Fear*. Revised and updated ed. New York: Warner Books.

Sadigh, M. 2001. *Autogenic Training: A Mind-Body Approach to the Treatment of Fibromyalgia and Chronic Pain Syndrome*. Binghamton, NY: Haworth Press.

Schultz, J. H., and W. Luthe. 1969. *Autogenic Therapy*. Vol. 1 of *Autogenic Methods*. New York: Grune and Stratton.

Recording

McManus, C. 2003. *Progressive Relaxation and Autogenic Training* (Audio CD). Produced by Carolyn McManus.

CHAPTER 10

Brief Combination Techniques

In this chapter you will learn to:

- Tailor relaxation techniques to fit your specific needs
- Combine techniques for a more powerful effect

Background

The relaxation exercises presented in this chapter are based on the work of many different therapists. They are creative blends of some of the techniques you've already learned. Learning several brief combination techniques can greatly benefit you for three reasons:

1. When you put two or more relaxation approaches together, the combination can have a *synergistic* effect. This means that the sum relaxation effect of the combined techniques is far greater than what you would achieve if you did each relaxation procedure individually. As you experiment with the material presented in this chapter, you'll learn which techniques are best at activating each other and combining for the most powerful effect.

2. The second reason that combining techniques is often more powerful than using one technique by itself is that the sequence of the combination is structured to draw you deeper into the relaxation experience. Each technique builds progressively on the one before. For example, the relaxation you experience from visualizing a pleasant beach scene is more profound if you precede the visualization with some deep breathing. And if you follow the deep breathing and the beach scene with autogenic themes of heaviness and warmth, you have a sequence of techniques that builds one upon the other to activate a deeper relaxation response.

3. The third advantage to using the combination techniques presented here is their brevity. You can easily do any of these combined sequences during a ten-minute coffee break. Any

time you have a few minutes to spare, these techniques can help you center yourself and regain a sense of calmness.

The combination techniques presented here are merely suggestions. Although each one has been tested and proven useful, feel free to be inventive. Try your own unique combinations. Experiment with a different sequence. Because you are a unique person with unique needs and patterns of responses, it's important for you to add, delete, and modify until you have a brief combined relaxation sequence that really works for you.

Symptom-Relief Effectiveness

The brief combination techniques presented here have been proven effective in the treatment of fight-or-flight symptoms and stress-induced physiological disorders. They are particularly helpful when your stress is work-related and requires brief but frequent booster sessions during the day to help you cope with mounting tensions.

Time to Master

If you have mastered the component techniques presented in earlier chapters, these combination approaches can be immediately and effectively applied. Otherwise, allow one to two weeks to use these combined approaches successfully.

Instructions

1. Stretch and Relax

A. While sitting in a chair, take a big stretch. Tighten your arms and pull them back so that you stretch your chest and shoulders. Stretch and tighten your legs at the same time by first pulling your toes up toward your knees and then pushing them out straight again.

B. Place one hand on your abdomen, just above your natural waist (where a belt would be most comfortable). Inhale slowly and deeply through your nose into your abdomen. Allow your hand to be pushed out by your exhale as much as feels comfortable. Take four more deep breaths using the same procedure.

C. Take hold of a pencil and suspend it by its point over a desk or table or the floor. Tell yourself that when you are deeply relaxed, the pencil will drop. The sound of the dropping pencil will be your signal to enter a healing five-minute trance. (If you prefer, you may omit the pencil and proceed with step C from here.) Close your eyes and say to yourself the key word or phrase that you've found most helpful in self-hypnosis. Tell yourself you will become more and more relaxed with each number as you count backward from ten to zero. After the countdown, repeat to yourself these four phrases, over and over, in any order: "I am drifting deeper and deeper, deeper and deeper.... I am more and more drowsy, peaceful, and calm.... I am drifting and drowsy, drowsy and drifting.... I am drifting down, down, down into total relaxation." If, by this time, your pencil has not already dropped, let go of it deliberately and remind yourself that you will now enjoy five minutes of peaceful self-hypnosis.

D. While in trance, visit your special place and enjoy the uniquely relaxing qualities of that environment. Really experience the sights, sounds, and sensations of your own special place. When it feels that you've been there long enough, count up from one to ten. Suggest to yourself that you are becoming more and more alert, refreshed, and wide awake as you count.

2. Abdominal Breathing and Imagination

This exercise combines the relaxing benefits of complete natural breathing with the curative value of positive autosuggestion.

A. Lie down on the floor on a rug or blanket in a dead-body pose (see description under Preparing to Do Breathing Exercises in chapter 3).

B. Place your hands gently on your solar plexus (the point where your ribs start to separate above your abdomen) and practice complete natural deep breathing for a few minutes.

C. Imagine energy is rushing into your lungs with each incoming breath of air and being immediately stored in your solar plexus. Imagine that this energy is flowing out to all parts of your body with each exhalation. Form a mental picture of this energizing process.

D. Continue doing this exercise on a daily basis for at least five to ten minutes a day.

3. Autogenic Breathing

A. Begin by taking slow, deep abdominal breaths as described in step 1B above. Become aware of your growing feeling of relaxation as each deep breath expands your diaphragm.

B. Visualize a beach. See the waves rolling up the sand, the seagulls wheeling overhead, a few puffs of fleecy clouds. Hear the roar of waves and then the quiet. Hear the alternating roar, quiet, roar, quiet. Over the ocean sound you can hear the seagulls calling. Now feel the warm sand. Imagine it covering your body, warm and heavy. Really feel the weight of the sand on your arms and legs. Feel surrounded by warmth and comfort.

C. While visualizing the sand, continue to breathe as deeply as feels comfortable. Notice the rhythm of your breath. As you breathe in, say the word "warm" to yourself. Try to feel the warmth of the sand around your body. As you breathe out, say the word "heavy." Experience the weight of the sand on your limbs. Continue your deep breathing, thinking *warm* as you inhale and *heavy* as you exhale. Continue for at least five minutes. (Note: If after a time you feel more comfortable shifting to shallower breathing, allow yourself to do so.)

4. I Am Grateful

This exercise is particularly helpful as the day is wearing on and your sense of stress and frustration is rising. It is also an excellent sequence for relaxing and putting yourself in a pleasant frame of mind before you drift off to sleep.

A. Use these steps from the Shorthand Procedure for progressive muscle relaxation outlined in chapter 4: (1) Curl fists, tighten biceps. Relax. (2) Wrinkle forehead and face like a walnut. Relax. (3) Arch back, and take a deep breath. Relax. (4) Pull feet back, curl toes while tightening calves, thighs, buttocks. Relax.

B. Reflect on the events of your day so far, and select three things for which you feel grateful. These don't have to be major events. For example, you may be grateful for the warm shower you took this morning, a coworker helping you with a difficult project, your child giving you a hug and telling you she loves you, a lovely sunrise, and so on. Take a moment to relive and enjoy these experiences.

C. Continue to think back over your day. Recall three things you did that you feel good about. Remember, these don't have to be major feats. For example, you may feel good about saying no to something you really didn't want to do, taking time for yourself to exercise or relax, or being supportive to someone you like. Take a minute to reexperience those positive moments.

5. Deep Affirmation

A. Put your hand over your abdomen and begin taking slow, deep abdominal breaths, as described in step 1B above.

B. Close your eyes and continue to breathe deeply as you scan your body for tension. Start with your toes and move up your body. Notice any tension in your calves, thighs, and buttocks. Explore areas of tension in your back, abdomen, or chest muscles. Notice your shoulders and neck, your jaw, cheeks, and forehead. Check for tension in your biceps, forearms, and hands. Whenever you discover a tense area, exaggerate the tension slightly so that you can become more aware of it. Notice exactly which muscles in your body are tense and then say to yourself, *I am tensing my* [insert the name of the muscle you're working with]. *I am hurting myself...I am creating tension in my body...I will let go of that tension starting now.*

C. Use the self-hypnosis exercise outlined in step 1C.

D. Select an affirmation to use while in trance. (The following list of suggested affirmations is reprinted with permission from *Visualization for Change* [1994] by Patrick Fanning.)

I can relax at will.

Tension is draining from my muscles.

I'm filled with peace, calm, and serenity.

I can turn my tension down like the volume on a radio.

Relaxation floods my body like healing, golden light.

I am in touch with my peaceful center.

I can look inward and find peace.

Relaxation is always within my grasp.

E. When you have relaxed long enough, count back up from one to ten. Suggest to yourself while you count that you are feeling more and more refreshed, alert, and wide awake.

6. The Tension Cutter

A. Take four deep abdominal breaths as described in step 1B.

B. Close your eyes. Visualize your tension by giving it a color and a shape. Now change the shape and color of your tension. Make it bigger or smaller, lighter or darker. Now see it moving farther and farther away from you. Watch it as it becomes smaller and smaller until it finally disappears from your awareness.

C. Now imagine your body filled with lights. See red lights for tension spots and blue lights for relaxed areas. Imagine the lights changing from red to blue in all the tension spots of your body. Be aware of any physical sensation you experience while you change to the blue light of relaxation. See all the lights in your body as blue and see the color blue becoming darker and darker. Feel yourself relaxing more deeply with each darker shade of blue you experience.

D. Now it's time for a mini-vacation. Here are two itineraries: pick one to enjoy or use them as a model for creating your own mini-vacation.

Vacation 1. Picture yourself in a forest. The light is clear and bright in places and dappled in others. As you take a long pleasant walk, you feel safe and comfortable. The air around you is cool and refreshing. You enjoy the bright spots of sunshine on the ground where sunlight filters down through the leaves. You are walking barefooted. The fallen leaves and moss feel soft and cool to your feet. You hear birdsong and the soft rustle of wind through the trees. These sounds make you feel happy and comfortable. As you walk, your muscles feel looser and looser, heavier, and more relaxed. The forest carpet of leaves and moss feels so comfortable that you want to lie down on it and close your eyes to rest. Now you see a small stream. It is making a soft, bubbly noise. Next to the stream is a patch of tall, soft grass, lit and warmed by sunlight. It's a lovely place to rest, and you sink down to your knees and roll gently over onto the soft, warm grass. You hear the bubbling stream, the birdsong, and the gentle wind. You are so deeply relaxed that every part of your body from your toes to the top of your head is loose and heavy.

Vacation 2. Picture yourself alone in a beach house with a view of the sea. The first rays of the morning sun light up the wall of your bedroom as you sink deeper into the warm, soft bed. You take a deep breath and notice how relaxed your muscles are. Outside you hear the sounds of seagulls and the rhythmic crashing of the waves. The waves roll in and out, in and out. Each wave makes you more and more deeply relaxed. In and out, in and out. You feel drowsy, heavy, and calm. You can feel the cool salt air coming through the open window, and you roll over to see the sand and the waves and the blue sky. You take deep breaths of the air, and your relaxation deepens with each breath. You feel safe and yet very free, unhurried, aware that the day ahead is full of possibilities.

7. Taking Control

A. Get comfortable, close your eyes, and begin noticing your breathing. Try to notice each breath and nothing else. As you exhale, say to yourself the word "one." Keep saying *one* with each exhalation.

B. When you feel sufficiently relaxed, turn your attention from your breathing to a situation you find stressful or difficult. See yourself handling that stressful situation confidently and successfully. See yourself saying and doing the appropriate thing to succeed. See yourself smiling, standing, or sitting erectly. Now visualize yourself hesitating or making a small error, uncertain for a moment. But then you recover, you go on, confidently finishing the task, looking satisfied. You remind yourself, *I can handle this. I'm in control.*

8. Accepting Yourself

A. Use the Body Scanning exercise from chapter 2 to become aware of how you are feeling in your body right now and what stressors might be contributing to how you feel.

B. Use abdominal breathing as described in step 1B to let go of the tension in your body and relax.

C. When you feel relaxed, make these suggestions to yourself: "I let go of shoulds… I accept myself with all my faults and weaknesses…. I breathe, I feel, I do the best I can." Rewrite this mantra in any manner that feels more authentic or true for you. Anything will work, as long as it carries the basic message that you accept yourself.

We also recommend that you review and consider incorporating the following techniques from these other chapters into your daily routine:

1. Mindful Breath Counting from chapter 3

2. Cue-Controlled Relaxation from chapter 7

3. Creating Your Special Place from chapter 6

Further Reading

Fanning, P. 1994. *Visualization for Change*. 2nd ed. Oakland, CA: New Harbinger Publications.

Recordings

Fanning, P., and M. McKay. 2008. *Daily Relaxer* (Audio CD). Oakland, CA: New Harbinger Publications.

Miller, E. 2003. *Letting Go of Stress* (Audio CD). Nevada City, CA: Emmett Miller. http://www.drmiller .com.

CHAPTER 11

Self-Compassion

In this chapter you will learn to:

- Feel compassion for yourself instead of judging yourself

- Increase your sense of well-being by accepting your failings and imperfections

Background

Your own opinion of yourself can be a significant source of stress in your life. When you feel that you are less than others and that you constantly fail to measure up, then life becomes a struggle. Your efforts to live up to the high standards you set for yourself create muscular tension and can lead to anxiety, depression, and anger.

In our competitive society it's all too easy to compare yourself to others and to feel that your self-worth depends on being above average in all things. This constant effort to pump up your self-esteem is exhausting and ultimately futile. Everybody in the world cannot be above average. Even if you are a high achiever in many realms, that is no guarantee of happiness.

Researcher Kristin Neff at the University of Texas at Austin has found that you're much better off if you abandon the pursuit of self-esteem and cultivate an attitude of loving-kindness toward yourself. In her book *Self-Compassion*, Neff tells the story of how she combined Buddhist mindfulness, her clinical psychology training, and her experiences in raising an autistic son into a series of exercises to increase self-compassion. At the University of Derby in the United Kingdom, professor Paul Gilbert has developed compassionate mind training (CMT), a group approach to increasing self-compassion. Both these researchers have found that seeking to build your self-esteem is a trickster trap that leads to stress and unhappiness. Compassion for yourself and others is a shorter road to relaxation and well-being.

Symptom-Relief Effectiveness

Self-compassion can reduce feelings of low self-worth, envy of the good fortune of others, and depression caused by an overly self-critical opinion of your abilities and traits. It provides relief from the anxiety of comparing yourself to others and increases both your acknowledgment of your strong points and your acceptance of your shortcomings and disappointments. Self-compassion will also help curb the anger you feel toward yourself for not measuring up to your own or others' expectations of you.

Time to Master

You can achieve some symptom relief immediately upon beginning self-compassion exercises. More profound and lasting results will come after you have been practicing self-compassion for a couple of months.

Building Self-Compassion

Self-compassion is a habit of thought and action. The best way to acquire this new habit is to try each of the exercises in this section. When you have that experience under your belt, you can then choose which exercises you might make part of a longer term or even daily practice.

A Compassionate Letter to Yourself

1. Use the form that follows to write a compassionate letter to yourself. This letter is going to be from the point of view of an imaginary friend who loves you, no matter what. (If this fill-in-the-blanks approach feels too constrained, write your letter on a blank sheet of paper, which will give you room to organize your thoughts and feelings more freely.)

2. Each section of the letter starts with one of the things that you don't like about yourself: your physical appearance, your bad habits, past actions or experiences you regret, and so on. Fill in the blanks with the things that make you feel inadequate or less than others.

3. After each issue, write how you feel about it: *ashamed*, *scared*, *regretful*, *depressed*, *angry*, *frustrated*, or any other feeling word that comes to mind.

4. Now the important part, the "however" section. This is where you take on the persona of an imaginary friend who always has your back. Write from the point of view of someone who feels nothing but deep compassion for you. No matter what you do, this person forgives. No matter how many times you fail or mess up, this person still loves you. This person wants you to succeed and thrive, but there is no pressure; there is just complete and utter acceptance.

Dear (your name) _____:

I know that when (your first issue) _____

_____ happens,

you feel (emotions) _____

_____.

However, _____

_____

_____.

And I know that when (your second issue) _____

_____ happens,

you feel (emotions) _____

_____.

However, _____

_____

_____.

And I know that when (your third issue) _____

_____ happens,

you feel (emotions) _____

_____.

However, _____

_____

_____.

Love,

Your friend forever

When you finish your letter, put it away for a few hours or a day. Then pull it out and read it. Dwell on the words and their meaning. Let the positive message fill you and relax the chronic tension of self-judgment. Tell yourself that you deserve this kind of all-accepting compassion.

Charlene was a single mom who clerked in a grocery store. She was stressed about money, her weight, and her daughter's drinking. Here is the compassionate letter that Charlene wrote herself:

Dear *Charlene*:

I know that when *you think about your daughter's drinking problem and her divorce*, you feel *responsible, like it is all somehow your fault and you should have done something different in raising her.*

However, *I also know that you were always doing your best in some hard situations. At any time in your daughter's life, you did what seemed right at the time, considering the circumstances and resources you had then. So you need to let it go and admit that you can't be responsible for another person that way.*

And I know that when *you look in the mirror and see the extra weight you've put on over the years*, you feel *ashamed and embarrassed about how you look.*

However, *that is just the surface reality. I know you deep down to the core. I know the caring, loving, sincere person you are. How you look is insignificant compared to who you are.*

And I know that when *you see Angela and Dawn, who have less seniority than you, promoted to assistant manager over your head*, you feel *angry about being passed over and depressed about your lack of advancement.*

However, *I admire how you have worked steadily since you were a teenager, putting a roof over your family's heads and bread on the table through good times and bad. You don't have any real control over who gets promoted at work, so no need to take it personally. If you just keep on keeping on, you can be proud of a job well done.*

Love,

Your friend forever

Way back in 1910, the French pharmacist and psychologist Emil Coué opened a clinic, where he told people to repeat to themselves, "Every day, in every way, I am getting better and better." Ever since, psychologists and self-improvement gurus have been recommending positive affirmations as a way to improve well-being. For much longer, Hindus and Buddhists have used *mantras*, words or sounds repeated, to aid concentration in meditation.

Kristin Neff (2011) recommends composing a personal mantra that reminds you of three things: that you are suffering, that suffering is normal, and that you can comfort yourself. Her personal mantra is "This is a moment of suffering. Suffering is part of life. May I be kind to myself in this moment. May I give myself the compassion I need" (119).

Self-Compassion Mantra

Compose your own mantra, in your own words, covering these three points in a way that makes sense to you:

1. I am suffering _____.

2. Suffering is inevitable _____.

3. I can comfort myself _____.

Melissa was a busy account executive and mother of two who had trouble getting out of the house on time in the morning. When her boys were fighting with each other instead of eating breakfast and getting their school stuff together, Melissa leaned against the refrigerator for a moment and recited her personal mantra to herself:

I'm struggling now, in this moment.

All life is a struggle.

Still, I love and cherish myself and my life.

Serenity...serenity.

A mantra does not have to sound like a prayer or a greeting card. Roger was a plainspoken heating and air-conditioning installer who got very tense and irritable by the end of a long day in the field. When he was behind schedule, lying on his back under a leaky compressor on a windy rooftop, he soothed himself with this self-compassion mantra he had composed for himself:

This is the shits.

Shit happens.

I can unclench and let it pass through me.

Softening Your Negatives

Fill in the blanks:

- A negative trait that I think defines me: _____

- I display this trait _____ percent of the time.

- I display this trait especially under these circumstances (family history, traumas, stresses):

  _____

  _____

- I have this trait because of these influences in my background:

  _____

  _____

If you're like most people, the first statement of your negative trait will be similar to Carol's:

- A negative trait that I think defines me: *I'm very critical of others.*

- I display this trait *40* percent of the time.

- I display this trait especially under these circumstances: *at work when incompetent people screw up.*

- I have this trait because of these influences in my background: *hypercritical parents, very competitive school.*

Ask yourself the following three questions and then rewrite your self-description:

1. When you are not displaying this negative trait, are you the same person?

2. When the triggering circumstances are not present and you are not displaying your negative trait, who are you then?

3. Are you entirely to blame for having this negative trait, considering your genetic makeup, early family upbringing, and the unavoidable traumas of life?

In light of these questions, reframe your self-description: _____

_____

_____

When Carol did the previous exercise, she was able to rewrite her self-description like this:

Since I am not hypercritical 60 percent of the time, it doesn't make sense to define my whole self as "very critical." In many situations—with my best friend, in my volunteer work, when I take my walks—I am not critical of others at all. Given how my parents were and the school I went to, it's entirely reasonable that I should have high standards for performance and low patience for inefficiency.

Self-Compassion Journal

Keep a self-compassion journal for a week.

1. Once a day, perhaps before bedtime, write down the most distressing experience you have had that day.

2. Include what happened, how you felt, your thoughts, and what, if anything, you did in response.

3. Conclude with a compassionate response to the memory that recognizes three facts: that you are only human, that you can be mindful of pain and let it pass, and that you can be kind to yourself.

Here are two daily entries from Ricardo's self-compassion journal. Ricardo was an apartment building manager in a high-rise full of demanding tenants. He recently was divorced from his wife Sally, and he missed his two young daughters.

Saturday: Mrs. Arcadian in 604 blew up her microwave by running it for an hour with nothing in it. Then she blames me for installing unsafe appliances! I felt furious at this stupid woman and yet guilty that I somehow had failed to warn her this could happen. I told myself that this kind of thing doesn't happen in a well-run building and that I should be able to prevent it. I was very curt and dismissive with Mrs. Arcadian.

I need to remember that I am only human, that I can only do my best at the moment. Remember that this too will pass. Remember that I love myself and forgive myself.

Sunday: Sally was an hour late dropping off the girls, so we missed the movie we wanted to see. Had to go to a later show, and then dinner was so late, they were cranky and horrible. I blew up at Sally in front of the girls, then was grouchy all evening. I felt angry and am now depressed at how our family has fallen apart. I blame myself a lot.

Sally and I and the girls are only human. We are going to make mistakes, and will have to fix them as best we can. I accept that these things happen, and we will get through them. I now choose to let go of all blaming—blaming Sally, blaming the girls, especially blaming myself.

Acts of Loving-Kindness Toward Yourself

Once a day, for the next week, do something kind and soothing for yourself. Pick something that you would not normally do: a special treat.

- Take a short walk in the park.

- Listen to a favorite song with your eyes closed; doing nothing but listening. Apply moisturizer or give yourself a foot rub.

- Sit in the yard with a cup of tea or a glass of wine.

- Stop in at an art gallery or museum.

- Avoid the kind of vices or indulgences that might make you feel guilty later, such as bingeing on food, drugging, or drinking.

This special treat serves as a reminder that it is right and good to feel for yourself the same compassion and loving-kindness that you might feel toward someone else in your place.

Final Thoughts

Remember that self-compassion is a habit of both thought and action. First you develop the habit of reminding yourself that you are not perfect, that you are as prone to mistakes as any other human being, and that you can forgive yourself for shortcomings and move on. Then you form the habit of self-care, taking the time you need to relax, to soothe yourself, and to enjoy the legitimate comforts and pleasures of life you deserve.

Further Reading

Gilbert, P. 2009. *The Compassionate Mind.* London: Constable.

Neff, K. 2011. *Self-Compassion: The Proven Power of Being Kind to Yourself.* New York: HarperCollins.

CHAPTER 12

Refuting Irrational Ideas

In this chapter you will learn to:

- Recognize how your thoughts influence your feelings, physical sensations, and behavior

- Assess your distressing thoughts

- Counteract your needless distressing thoughts

Background

Almost every minute of your conscious life, you are engaging in *self-talk*, your internal thought language. These are the sentences with which you describe and interpret the world. If your self-talk is accurate and in touch with reality, you function well. If it is irrational and untrue, you experience stress and emotional disturbance. Here is an example of irrational self-talk: *I can't bear to be alone.* No physically healthy person has ever died merely from being alone. Being alone may be uncomfortable, undesirable, and frustrating, but you can live with it and live through it.

Another example of irrational self-talk might be *I should never be cruel to my child. If I am, I'll know I'm a rotten person.* The phrase "should never" allows no possibility of flaw or failure. When the inevitable quarrel occurs, you indict yourself as entirely rotten—all on the basis of a single incident.

Irrational ideas may be based on outright misperceptions ("When the airplane's wing shakes, I know it's going to fall off") or the perfectionist's *shoulds*, *oughts*, and *musts* ("I ought to keep quiet rather than risk upsetting anyone"). Inaccurate self-talk such as "I need love" is emotionally dangerous compared to the more realistic "I want love very much, but I don't absolutely need it, and can survive and feel reasonably happy without it." "How terrible to be rejected" is fear producing in comparison to "I find it unpleasant, awkward in the moment, and feel regretful when I am rejected." Imperatives such as "I've got to be more helpful around the house" can be converted to more rational statements, such as "There would probably be more peace and compatibility in my home if I did a greater share of the work."

Albert Ellis developed a system to attack irrational ideas or beliefs and replace them with realistic statements about the world. He called his system "rational emotive therapy" and wrote about it, with coauthor Robert Harper, in *A Guide to Rational Living* (1975) first published in 1961. Ellis's basic thesis is that emotions are only partially related to actual events. Between the event and the emotion is realistic or unrealistic self-talk. The self-talk produces the emotions. Your own thoughts, directed and controlled by you, are what create anxiety, anger, and depression. Ellis later renamed his system "rational emotive behavior therapy," stressing that people's actions as well as their emotions are influenced by their ideas. The image below shows how it works.

Feedback Loop

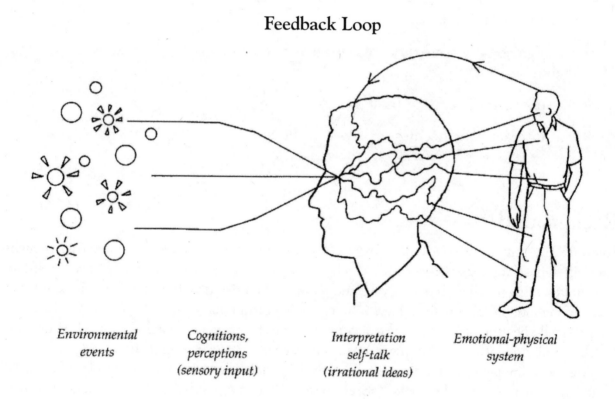

| Environmental events | Cognitions, perceptions (sensory input) | Interpretation self-talk (irrational ideas) | Emotional-physical system |

Example

Ellis's model is as simple as A, B, C:

Activating Facts and Events

A mechanic replaces a fuel pump he honestly believes was malfunctioning, but the car's performance doesn't improve. The customer is very upset and demands that the mechanic put the old fuel pump back.

Beliefs or Negative Self-Talk About Activating Facts or Event

The mechanic says to himself,

He's just a grouch—nothing would please him.

and

Why the hell do I get all the tough jobs?

and

I ought to have figured this out by now.

and, finally,

I'm not much of a mechanic.

Consequences: Emotions, Sensations, and Behavior

The mechanic feels anger, resentment, and depression, as well as a sense of worthlessness. He feels a knot in his stomach. As the day wears on, he develops a headache. He reluctantly agrees to put in the old fuel pump, but for the rest of the day he is short-tempered with coworkers and then with his family later that night.

The mechanic may later say to himself, *That guy really made me mad.* But it is not the customer or anything the customer has done that produces the anger—it is the mechanic's own self-talk, his interpretation of reality. Such irrational self-talk can be changed and the stressful emotions, sensations, and behavior that result from this self-talk can be changed with it.

Symptom-Relief Effectiveness

Rimm and Litvak (1969) found that negative self-talk produced substantial physiological arousal. In other words, your body tenses and becomes stressed when you use irrational arguments such as:

People seem to ignore me at parties.

$\downarrow$

It's obvious that I'm either boring or unattractive to them.

$\downarrow$

How terrible!

The emotional results of irrational negative self-talk are anxiety, depression, rage, guilt, jealousy, low frustration tolerance, shame, and a sense of worthlessness. Rational emotive behavior therapy has been shown to be effective in decreasing the frequency and intensity of these emotions.

Time to Master

Assessment of your irrational beliefs, plus homework sufficient to refute one of these beliefs, can take approximately twenty minutes a day for two weeks. Rational emotive imagery, the process by which you work directly on changing your emotions, also takes about two weeks if you practice ten minutes a day.

Instructions

Beliefs Inventory

The following Beliefs Inventory will help you uncover some of the irrational ideas that contribute to unhappiness and stress. Take the test now, score it, and note the sections where your scores are highest.

Note that it is not necessary to think over any item very long. Mark your answer quickly and go on to the next statement. Be sure to mark how you actually think about the statement, not how you think you should think.

Beliefs Inventory

Somewhat Agree	Agree	Disagree	Score	Belief
	√		2	1. It is important to me that others approve of me.
	√		2	2. I hate to fail at anything.
√			A	3. People who do wrong deserve what they get.
√			A	4. When I don't get what I want, I get mad.
		√	0	5. Negative feelings are natural consequences of negative events.

	√		2	6. I need everyone to like me.
	√		2	7. I avoid things I cannot do well.
	√	√	0	8. Too many bad people escape the punishment they deserve.
√			∧	9. I'm easily frustrated when things don't go my way.
√			∧	10. The best way to avoid pain and be happy is to have control over your environment.
		√	0	11. I find it hard to go against what others think.
	√		2	12. It is very important to me to be successful in everything I do.
	√		2	13. Those who do wrong deserve to be blamed and punished.
	√		2	14. I often get disturbed over situations I don't like.
		√	0	15. People who are miserable are victims of circumstances beyond their control.
	√		2	16. I often worry about how much people approve of and accept me.
	√		2	17. It upsets me a lot when I make mistakes.
√			∧	18. Immorality should be strongly punished.
		√	0	19. I get extremely annoyed when others inconvenience me.
		√	0	20. The more problems a person has, the less happy he or she will be.
	√		2	21. I worry a lot about what people think about me.
	√		2	22. I'm afraid to do things that I cannot do well.
		√	0	23. I hold grudges against people who have wronged me.
		√	0	24. Things should be different than the way they are.
		√	0	25. Inconsiderate people annoy the heck out of me.
	√		2	26. I often can't get my mind off some concern.
	√		2	27. I usually put off important decisions.
		√	0	28. Everyone needs someone he or she can depend on for help and advice.

		√	0	29. It is almost impossible to overcome the influences of the past.
		√	0	30. To be happy, I would need a lifelong leisurely vacation.
		√	0	31. I can't stand to take chances.
√			ʌ	32. I avoid facing my problems.
		√	0	33. People absolutely need a source of strength outside themselves.
		√	0	34. If I had had different experiences, I could be more like the person I want to be.
		√	0	35. I feel most content when I have nothing to do.
√			ʌ	36. I worry a lot about certain things in the future.
	√		2	37. I often put things off.
		√	0	38. There are certain people upon whom I greatly depend.
	√		2	39. I often think of past experiences as affecting me now.
√			ʌ	40. I prefer quiet leisure above all things.
		√	0	41. I feel anxious when I think about unexpected dangers or future events.
	√		2	42. It is difficult for me to do unpleasant chores even if they benefit me.
		√	0	43. I must always seek the advice of others before making any important decision.
		√	0	44. Once something strongly affects your life, it always will.
		√	0	45. It is only through leisure and relaxation that I can find fulfillment.
		√	0	46. If something happened that I was afraid of, it would be terrible, and I couldn't stand it.
√			ʌ	47. I dislike responsibility and avoid it if I can.
		√	0	48. I need people in my life whom I can rely upon to feel safe.
		√	0	49. People never change basically.
		√	0	50. I shouldn't have to work at being happy.

Scoring the Beliefs Inventory:

- Give the items you marked as "disagree" a score of 0, items you marked as "somewhat agree" a score of 1, and items you marked as "agree" a score of 2.

- Add up your points for items 1, 6, 11, 16, and 21, and enter the total here: __8__. The higher the total, the more you agree with the irrational idea that *It is an absolute necessity for an adult to have love and approval from peers, family, and friends.*

- Add up your points for items 2, 7, 12, 17, and 22, and enter the total here: __10__. The higher the total, the more you agree with the irrational idea that *You must be unfailingly competent and almost perfect in all you undertake.*

- Add up your points for items 3, 8, 13, 18, and 23, and enter the total here: __4__. The higher the total, the more you agree with the irrational idea that *Certain people are evil, wicked, and villainous and should be punished.*

- Add up your points for items 4, 9, 14, 19, and 24, and enter the total here: __4__. The higher the total, the more you agree with the irrational idea that *It is horrible when things are not the way you would like them to be.*

- Add up your points for items 5, 10, 15, 20, and 25, and enter the total here: __1__. The higher the total, the more you agree with the irrational idea that *External events cause most human misery—that people simply react as events trigger their emotions.*

- Add up your points for items 26, 31, 36, 41, and 46, and enter the total here: __3__. The higher the total, the more you agree with the irrational idea that *You should feel fear or anxiety about anything that is unknown, uncertain, or potentially dangerous.*

- Add up your points for items 27, 32, 37, 42, and 47, and enter the total here: __8__. The higher the total, the more you agree with the irrational idea that *It is easier to avoid than face life's difficulties and responsibilities.*

- Add up your points for items 28, 33, 38, 43, and 48, and enter the total here: __0__. The higher the total, the more you agree with the irrational idea that *You need something other or stronger or greater than yourself to rely upon.*

- Add up your points for items 29, 34, 39, 44, and 49, and enter the total here: __2__. The higher the total, the more you agree with the irrational idea that *The past has a lot to do with determining the present.*

- Add up your points for items 30, 35, 40, 45, and 50, and enter the total here: __1__. The higher the total, the more you agree with the irrational idea that *Happiness can be achieved by inaction, passivity, and endless leisure.*

Irrational Ideas

At the root of all irrational thinking is the assumption that things are done to you: *That really got me down... She makes me nervous... Places like that scare me... Being lied to makes me see red.* Nothing is done to you. Events happen in the world. You experience those activating events (A), engage in self-talk (B), and consequently experience an emotion (C) resulting from the self-talk. A does not cause C; B causes C. If your self-talk is irrational and unrealistic, you create unpleasant emotions.

Two common forms of irrational self-talk are statements that *awfulize* and *absolutize*. You awfulize by making catastrophic, nightmarish interpretations of your experience. A momentary chest pain is a heart attack, the grumpy boss intends to fire you, your spouse takes a night job and the thought of being alone is unthinkably terrible. Awfulizing involves exaggerating unwanted events, traits, or behaviors while almost always ignoring the positive ones. The emotions that follow awfulizing self-talk tend themselves to be awful—you are responding to your own description of the world.

For instance, if you think that a situation is painful, boring, or difficult and you exaggerate these qualities beyond your ability to cope, you'd likely feel overwhelmed. If you define people by their flaws or misdeeds and tell yourself these flaws or misdeeds are horrible, they become terrible people. It becomes easy to justify your anger. Irrational self-statements that absolutize often include words like "should," "must," "ought," "always," and "never." The idea is that other people or things must be a certain way, or you must be a certain way. Any deviation from that particular value or standard is bad. The person who fails to live up to the standard is bad. In reality, the standard is what's bad, because it is inflexible and narrow-minded.

Irrational Ideas Checklist

Albert Ellis suggested ten basic irrational ideas, which are listed below. To these we have added some additional common self-statements that are highly unrealistic. Based on your scores on the Beliefs Inventory, and your knowledge of the situations in which you characteristically experience stress, place a check mark next to the ones that seem to apply to you.

_____✓_____ 1. **It is an absolute necessity for an adult to have love and approval from peers, family, and friends.** In fact, pleasing all the people in your life is impossible. Even those who basically like and approve of you will be turned off by some behaviors and qualities. This irrational belief is one of the greatest causes of misery.

_____✓_____ 2. **You must be unfailingly competent, successful, and almost perfect in all that you undertake.** The results of believing that you must behave perfectly are self-blame for inevitable failure, lowered self-esteem, perfectionistic standards applied to spouse and friends, and paralysis and fear at attempting anything. Compare this to the belief that you can strive to do your best and learn from your errors.

_____ 3. **Certain people are evil, wicked, and villainous and should be punished.** A more realistic position is that they are behaving in ways that are antisocial or inappropriate. They are perhaps stupid, ignorant, or neurotic and may need to change their behavior.

_____ 4. **It is horrible when people and things are not the way you would like them to be.** This might be described as the spoiled-child syndrome. As soon as the tire goes flat the self-talk starts: *Why does this happen to me? Damn, I can't take this. It's awful, I'll get all filthy.* Any inconvenience, problem, or failure to get your way is likely to be met with such awfulizing self-statements. The result is intense irritation and stress.

_____ 5. **External events cause most human misery—people simply react as events trigger their emotions.** A logical extension of this belief is that you must control external events in order to create happiness or avoid sorrow. The fact is, our control is limited and we are at a loss to completely manipulate the wills of others. Interpreting an event as the reason for your unhappiness can keep you stuck. Although you may have only limited control over others, you do have enormous control over your thoughts, emotions, and behavior.

✓   6. **You should feel fear or anxiety about anything that is unknown, uncertain, or potentially dangerous.** Many describe this as "a little bell goes off and I think I ought to start worrying." They begin to rehearse their catastrophe scenarios. Increasing the fear or anxiety in the face of uncertainty makes coping more difficult and adds to stress. Saving the fear response for actual, perceived danger allows you to enjoy uncertainty as a novel and exciting experience.

7. **It is easier to avoid than to face life's difficulties and responsibilities.** There are many ways of ducking responsibilities: *I should tell him I'm no longer interested—but not tonight… I'd like to get another job, but I'm just too tired on my days off to look… A leaky faucet won't hurt anything…* If this way of thinking applies to you, write down your standard excuses to avoid responsibility:

Area of Responsibility	Method of Avoidance
Replying to messages	I can do that later
telling people disappointing news	I still have time, now is not the right time
take big decisions	the solution will come to me
study	I will do it tomorrow

8. **You absolutely need something other or stronger or greater than yourself to rely upon.** This belief becomes a psychological trap in which your independent judgment and your awareness of your particular needs are undermined by a complete reliance on higher authority.

9. **The past has a lot to do with determining the present.** Just because you were once strongly affected by something does not mean that you must continue the habits you formed to cope with the original situation. Those old patterns and ways of responding are just decisions made so many times that they have become nearly automatic. You can identify those old decisions and start changing them right now. You can learn from past experience, but you don't have to be overly attached to it.

10. **Happiness can be achieved by inaction, passivity, and endless leisure.** This is called the Elysian Fields syndrome. There is more to happiness than perfect relaxation.

Other Irrational Ideas

_____ 1. **People are fragile and should never be hurt.** This irrational belief results in failure to openly communicate important feelings and in self-sacrifice that gives up what is nourishing and pleasurable (Farquhar and Lowe 1974). Because everything you want seems to hurt or deprive someone else, you feel frustration, helplessness, and depression. Relationships become full of dead space where conflicts have developed and nothing was said to resolve them.

_____ 2. **Good relationships are based on mutual sacrifice and a focus on giving.** This belief rests on the assumption that it is better to give than to receive. It is expressed in a reluctance to ask for what you want and need and the anticipation that your hidden needs will be divined and provided for. Unfortunately, constant self-denial usually results in bitterness and withdrawal.

___√___ 3. **If you don't go to great lengths to please others, they will abandon or reject you.** This belief is a by-product of low self-esteem. You usually run less risk of rejection if you offer others your true unembellished self. They can take it or leave it. However, if they get to know the real you, you don't have to worry about slacking off, letting down your guard, and being rejected later.

___√___ 4. **When people disapprove of you, it invariably means you are wrong or bad.** This extremely crippling belief sparks chronic anxiety in most interpersonal situations (Farquhar and Lowe 1974). The irrationality is contained in the generalization of one specific fault or unattractive feature to a total indictment of the self.

_____ 5. **Happiness, pleasure, and fulfillment can occur only in the presence of others, and being alone is horrible.** Pleasure, self-worth, and fulfillment can be experienced alone as well as with others (Farquhar and Lowe 1974). Being alone is growth producing and, at times, desirable.

___√___ 6. **There is perfect love and a perfect relationship.** Subscribers to this belief often feel dissatisfied and resentful of one close relationship after another. Nothing is quite right, because they are waiting for the perfect fit, which never comes.

_____ 7. **You shouldn't have to feel pain; you are entitled to a good life.** The realistic position is that pain is an inevitable part of human life. Pain frequently accompanies tough, healthy decisions and the process of growth. Life is not fair, and sometimes you will suffer no matter what you do.

_√_   8. **Your worth as a person depends on how much you achieve and produce.** A more rational assessment of your real worth would depend on such things as your capacity to experience being fully alive, feeling everything it means to be human (Farquhar and Lowe 1974).

_√_   9. **Anger is automatically bad and destructive.** Anger as an act is frequently cleansing and can be an honest communication of current feelings without attacking the personal worth and security of others (Farquhar and Lowe 1974).

_√_   10. **It is bad or wrong to be selfish.** The truth is that no one knows your needs and wants better than you, and no one else has as great an interest in seeing them fulfilled. Your happiness is your responsibility. Being selfish means you are accepting that responsibility. At the same time, you can respect others' right to take responsibility for their own happiness.

_____   11. **You are helpless and have no control over what you experience or feel.** This belief is at the heart of much depression and anxiety. In truth, we have some control over interpersonal situations and a lot of control over how we interpret and emotionally respond to life events.

You can add other irrational beliefs to this list:

_____

_____

_____

_____

_____

_____

Identifying Elusive Irrational Ideas

Much of the difficulty in uncovering irrational self-talk results from the speed and invisibility of thoughts. They may be lightning quick and barely on the edge of awareness. You will rarely be conscious of a complete sentence, as in the irrational statements above. Because self-talk has a reflexive, automatic quality, it is easy to keep the illusion that feelings arise spontaneously from events. However, once the thoughts are slowed down like a slow-motion film, frame by frame, the millisecond it takes to say "I'm falling apart" is exposed for its malignant influence. The thoughts that create your emotions frequently may appear in a kind of shorthand: *No good…crazy…feeling sick…dumb*, and so on. That shorthand has to be stretched out into the original sentence it was extracted from. The sentence can then be challenged with methods you'll learn in the next section on refuting irrational ideas.

The best way to uncover your irrational ideas is to reflect on situations in which you experience distressing emotions such as anxiety, depression, anger, guilt, or a sense of worthlessness. Behind each of these emotions, particularly if they are chronic, is irrational self-talk. Ask yourself, **What am I telling myself about this situation?** You may be tempted to immediately self-correct with rational self-talk. For instance, in response to the irrational thought *My brother never helps out with our elderly parents; it's just not fair*, Amy might have immediately told herself, *Nobody said life was fair*. This would have prevented her from exploring the other thoughts that are distressing her.

Instead, she asked herself, **What if that were true? What would it mean to me?** (Burns 1999). To this, she responded, *He has it easy. I want his easy life. I'm really as selfish as he is. But I have no right to be angry.* By repeatedly asking herself the three questions in bold type, Amy was able to identify many of her other upsetting, irrational thoughts, including these: *It's only right to sacrifice my life—after all, they're family. I love my parents, but they're driving me crazy! I should be stronger. I feel like I'm drowning. What if something happens to me—what will happen to them? I can't stand to think of them all alone. That would be a disaster.…* Amy wrote down these thoughts in a notebook to refer to later.

As you can probably imagine, Amy is in an objectively difficult situation. In addition, she has many irrational thoughts that are generating so much distress that she isn't able to problem solve effectively or to make sensible decisions. She can use the next technique to step back from and challenge the irrational ideas that are bothering her the most.

Refuting Irrational Ideas

There are five steps (A through E) to disputing and eliminating irrational ideas. Begin by selecting a situation that consistently generates stressful emotions in you.

A. **Write the facts** of the event as they occurred at the time you were upset. Be sure to include only the objective facts, not conjectures, subjective impressions, or value judgments.

B. **Write your self-talk** about the event. State all your subjective value judgments, assumptions, beliefs, predictions, and worries. Note which self-statements have been previously described as irrational ideas.

C. **Focus on your emotional response.** Make a clear one- or two-word label, such as "angry," "depressed," "felt worthless," "afraid," and so on.

D. **Dispute and change the irrational self-talk** identified in step B. Here's how it is done, according to Ellis:

1. **Select the irrational idea that you wish to dispute.** As an illustration, we will use the irrational idea "It's not fair that I have to suffer with such a problem."

2. **Is there any rational support for this idea?** Since everything is as it should be, given long chains of cause and effect, the answer is no. The problem must be endured and dealt with because it happened. It happened because all the conditions necessary to make it happen existed.

3. **What evidence exists for the falseness of this idea?**

   a. *There are no laws of the universe that say I should not have pain or problems. I can experience any problem for which the necessary conditions exist.*

   b. *Life is not fair. Life is just a sequence of events, some of which bring pleasure and some of which are inconvenient and painful.*

   c. *If problems occur, it is up to me to try to solve them.*

   d. *Trying to keep a problem from developing is adaptive, but resenting and not facing it once it exists is a dangerous strategy.*

   e. *No one is special. Some people go through life with relatively less pain than I do. This is due to one of two things: the luck of the draw or decisions I've made that contributed to the necessary conditions for my problems.*

   f. *Just because I have a problem doesn't mean I have to be miserable. I can take pride in the challenge of a creative solution. This may be an opportunity to increase my self-esteem.*

4. **Does any evidence exist for the truth of this idea?** *No, my suffering is due to my self-talk, how I have interpreted this event. I have convinced myself that I should be unhappy.*

5. **What is the worst thing that could happen to you** if what you want to happen doesn't, or what you don't want to happen does?

   a. *I could be deprived of various pleasures while I deal with the problem.*

   b. *I might feel inconvenienced.*

   c. *I might never solve the problem and experience myself as ineffective in this particular area.*

   d. *I might have to accept the consequences of failure.*

   e. *Others might not approve of how I am behaving or I might be rejected as incompetent.*

   f. *I might feel more stress and tension.*

6. **What good things might occur** if what you want to happen doesn't, or what you don't want to happen does?

   a. *I might learn to tolerate frustration better.*

   b. *I might improve my coping skills.*

   c. *I might become more responsible.*

E. **Substitute alternative self-talk,** now that you have clearly examined the irrational idea and compared it with rational thinking.

   1. *There's nothing special about me. I can accept painful situations when they emerge.*

   2. *Facing the problem is more adaptive than resenting it or running away from it.*

   3. *I feel what I think. If I don't think negative thoughts, I won't feel stressed out. At worst, I will experience inconvenience, regret, and annoyance—not anxiety, depression, and rage.*

Homework

To succeed in your war against irrational ideas, you need a daily commitment to doing homework. Download the blank Homework Sheet from http://www.newharbinger.com/43348 and make about a hundred copies to use after an activating event occurs; fill out the sheet at least once a day, spending at least twenty minutes on it. Whenever possible, do your homework right after the event. Use separate sheets for each event, and save them as a record of your growth.

First look at this sample homework completed by a man who had a date with a friend who canceled.

Sample Homework Sheet

A. **Activating event:**

A friend canceled a date with me.

B. **Rational ideas:**

I know she's under a lot of time pressure right now…I'll do something by myself.

Irrational ideas:

I'll feel terribly alone tonight… The emptiness is setting in… She doesn't really care for me… No one really wants to spend time with me… I'm falling apart.

C. **Consequences of the irrational ideas:**

I was depressed… I was moderately anxious.

D. **Disputing and challenging the irrational ideas:**

1. Select the irrational idea:

   I'll feel terribly alone tonight… I'm falling apart.

2. Is there any rational support for this idea?

   No.

3. What evidence exists for the falseness of the idea?

   Being alone is not as pleasurable as having a date, but I can find pleasure in an alternative activity.

   I usually enjoy being alone, and I will tonight as soon as I face the disappointment.

   I'm mislabeling frustration and disappointment as "falling apart."

4. Does any evidence exist for the truth of the idea?

   No, only that I've talked myself into feeling depressed.

5. What is the worst thing that could happen to me?

   I could continue to feel disappointed and not find anything really pleasurable to do tonight.

6. What good things might occur?

   I might feel more self-reliant and realize that I do have inner resources.

E. **Alternative thoughts:**

I'm okay. I'll get out my detective novel. I'll treat myself to a good Chinese dinner. I'm good at being alone.

Alternative emotions:

I feel quiet, a little disappointed, but I'm anticipating a good meal and a good book.

Homework Sheet

A. **Activating event:** _____

_____

B. **Rational ideas:** _____

_____

Irrational ideas: _____

_____

C. **Consequences of the irrational ideas:** _____

_____

D. **Disputing and challenging the irrational ideas:**

1. Select the irrational idea: _____

_____

2. Is there any rational support for this idea? _____

3. What evidence exists for the falseness of the idea? _____

_____

_____

4. Does any evidence exist for the truth of the idea? _____

_____

5. What is the worst thing that could happen to me? _____

_____

6. What good things might occur? _____

_____

E. **Alternative thoughts:** _____

_____

Alternative emotions: _____

_____

Rules to Promote Rational Thinking

Evaluate your self-statements against these six rules, or guidelines, for rational thinking (adapted from David Goodman's *Emotional Well-Being Through Rational Behavior Training* [1978]).

1. **It doesn't do anything to me.** The situation doesn't make me anxious or afraid. I say things to myself that largely produce my anxiety and fear.

2. **Everything is exactly the way it should be.** The conditions for things or people to be otherwise don't exist. To say that things should be other than what they are is to believe in magic. They are what they are because of a long series of causal events, including interpretations, responses from irrational self-talk, and so on. To say that things should be different is to throw out causality.

3. **All humans are fallible creatures.** This is inescapable. If you haven't set reasonable quotas of failure for yourself and others, you increase the prospects for disappointment and unhappiness. It becomes all too easy to attack yourself and others as worthless, bad, and so on.

4. **It takes two to have a conflict.** Before beginning a course of accusation and blame, consider the 30 percent rule. Any party to a conflict is contributing at least 30 percent of the fuel to keep it going.

5. **The original cause is lost in antiquity.** Trying to discover who did what first is a waste of time. The search for the original cause of chronic painful emotions is extremely difficult. The best strategy is to make decisions to change your behavior now.

6. **We largely feel the way we think.** This is the positively stated principle behind the first statement in this list. This statement reinforces the idea that events don't cause emotions—our interpretations of events cause emotions.

Special Considerations

If you have difficulty making headway with rational emotive behavior therapy, one of three factors may be influencing your difficulties:

1. You remain unconvinced that thoughts cause emotions. If this is the case, confine your work initially to rational emotive imagery, which is described next. If you then find that changes in your self-talk can push you toward experiencing less stressful emotions, the statement that thoughts cause emotions may become more believable.

2. Your irrational ideas and self-talk are so lightning-swift that you have difficulty catching them. If this is the case, try keeping a journal of events and situations associated with

intense emotions. Put down everything that flows through your mind: scenes, images, single words, vague half-formed thoughts, names, sounds, sentences, and so on.

3. You have difficulty remembering your thoughts. If this is the case, don't wait until after the fact. Use a journal to write everything down just as it is happening.

Rational Emotive Imagery

In 1971, Dr. Maxie Maultsby introduced rational emotive imagery. This technique will help you develop strategies to change stressful emotions. It works as follows:

1. Imagine an event that is stressful and usually accompanied by unpleasant emotions. Notice all the details of the situation: sights, smells, sounds, how you are dressed, what is being said, and so on.

2. As you clearly imagine the event, allow yourself to feel uncomfortable. Let in the emotions of anger, anxiety, depression, worthlessness, or shame. Don't try to avoid the emotion—go ahead and feel it.

3. After experiencing the stressful emotion, push yourself to change it to a healthier negative emotion. You can fundamentally alter these emotions so that anxiety, depression, rage, and guilt are replaced by keenly felt concern, disappointment, annoyance, or regret. If you think you can't do this, you are only fooling yourself. Everyone can change a feeling, if only for a few moments.

4. Having contacted the stressful feeling and pushed it, however briefly, into a healthier negative emotion, you can examine how you did it. What happened inside your head that altered your original depression, anxiety, or rage? Clearly, you told yourself something different about yourself, or others, or the situation.

5. Instead of saying "I can't handle this…this will drive me crazy," you might now be saying "I've dealt successfully with situations like this before." You have changed your beliefs, your interpretations of experience. Once you know how you changed the stressful emotion to a healthier negative emotion, you can substitute the new, adaptive beliefs any time you want. Become deeply aware of how the new beliefs lead you away from stress and produce more bearable emotions.

For example, a housewife, who became depressed whenever her husband turned on the television in the evening, practiced rational emotive imagery. During the day, she conjured up the situation in her imagination: her husband wiping his mouth, getting up from the table, taking the plates to the sink, and leaving the room. She could imagine a few moments later the sound of the television coming on, the changing of channels, the voices from his favorite sitcom. As she reviewed the sequence, she sank into despondency and became depressed.

After coming fully in contact with the stressful emotion, she pushed herself to change the feeling of depression into one of disappointment and irritation. This felt like shoving a huge rock single-handed. It took fifteen minutes of effort before she could get even momentary contact with the less stressful emotions. By practicing at hourly intervals, she was soon able to push her depression into irritation or disappointment for several minutes.

She became ready to examine how she had changed her thoughts (self-talk) in order to change her emotions. She found she could change depression into irritation by telling herself *I don't have to feel helpless. If he wants to spend his time with TV, I can do something that feels good to me.* Her other thoughts included: *It's his life. He can waste it if he wants to. I'm not going to waste mine. There are people I don't visit, because I think I should stay home with him. But I'm going to take care of myself. He may be displeased if I don't stay home, but staying home to watch the tube is not satisfying for me.*

Developing Alternative Emotional Responses

Here is a list of sample situations and alternative emotional responses:

Situation	Unhealthy Negative Emotion	Healthy Negative Emotion
Fight with mate	Rage	Annoyance, irritation
Work deadline	High anxiety	Concern
Cruelty to a child	Intense guilt	Regret
Something you enjoy is canceled	Depression	Disappointment
Criticized	Feeling worthless	Annoyance, concern
A public mistake	Shame	Guilt about your act, not self

Now fill in your own stressful situations, including the unhealthy negative emotions you feel and the healthier negative emotions you would like to feel.

Situation	Unhealthy Negative Emotion	Healthy Negative Emotion

You can use rational emotive imagery in each of these situations. If the unhealthy negative emotions do not change right away, let yourself keep feeling them until they do change. You *can* alter these emotions by merely pushing yourself to do so. Afterward, you will isolate the key thoughts and phrases that made the new, healthier emotions possible. Changing your self-talk to include these more adaptive thoughts, beliefs, and ideas will make it increasingly easy for you to change the emotion you're working with. For best results, practice this technique ten minutes a day for at least two weeks.

Insight

Understand that there are three levels of insight necessary for change to take place. They are the following:

1. Knowing that you have a problem, and awareness of some of the events that may have caused the problem.

2. Seeing clearly that the irrational ideas you acquired early in life are creating the emotional climate you live in now, and that consciously or unconsciously you work fairly hard to perpetuate those irrational ideas.

3. Believing strongly that after recognizing the validity of these two prior insights, you will still find no way to eliminate the problem other than working to change your irrational ideas, steadily, persistently, and vigorously.

Without making a commitment to this last insight, you will experience difficulties altering your habitual emotional responses.

If you think this technique could be useful to you but you are unable to master it, contact a rational emotive therapist or center for consultation.

Further Reading

Beck, A. T. 1989. *Love Is Never Enough: How Couples Can Overcome Misunderstandings, Resolve Conflict, and Solve Relationship Problems with Cognitive Therapy.* Reprint ed. New York: HarperCollins.

———. 2016. "Cognitive Therapy: Nature and Relation to Behavior Therapy." *Behavior Therapy* 47 (6): 776–84. (Originally published in 1970.)

Burns, D. D. 1999. *The Feeling Good Handbook.* Revised ed. New York: Penguin Books.

Ellis, A. 1980. *Growth Through Reason.* Palo Alto, CA: Science and Behavior Books.

———. 1986. *Anger: How to Live With and Without It.* New York: Carol Publishing Group.

———. 2001. *Overcoming Destructive Beliefs, Feelings, and Behaviors: New Directions for Rational Emotive Behavior Therapy.* Amherst, NY: Prometheus Books.

———. 2016. *Anger: How to Stubbornly Refuse to Make Yourself Miserable About Anything—Yes, Anything.* Revised ed. New York: Carol Publishing Group.

Ellis, A., and R. J. Harper. 1975. *A Guide to Rational Living.* 3rd ed. North Hollywood, CA: Wilshire Book Company.

Ellis, A., and C. MacLaren. 2005. *Rational Emotive Behavior Therapy: A Therapist's Guide.* 2nd ed. Atascadero, CA: Impact Publishers.

Farquhar, W., and J. Lowe. 1974. "A List of Irrational Ideas." In *Youth: Toward Personal Growth; A Rational Emotive Approach*, edited by D. J. Tosi. Columbus, OH: Charles E. Merrill.

Goodman, D. 1978. *Emotional Well-Being Through Rational Behavior Training.* Springfield, IL: Charles C. Thomas Publisher.

Lazarus, A. A. 1996. *Behavior Therapy and Beyond* (Master Work Series). New York: Jason Aronson.

Maultsby, M. 1971. "Rational Emotive Imagery." *Rational Living* 6 (1): 24–27.

Rimm, D. C., and S. B. Litvak. 1969. "Self-Verbalization and Emotional Arousal." *Journal of Abnormal Psychology* 74 (2): 181–87.

CHAPTER 13

Relieving Worry and Anxiety

In this chapter you will learn to:

- Use relaxation skills to reduce tension and arousal in general as well as in stressful situations

- Observe objectively the thoughts, feelings, and behaviors associated with anxiety

- Use the anxiety management skill of defusion to deal with worry thoughts

- Identify and change safety behaviors such as excessive checking and avoidance

- Solve problems effectively

Background

A little anxiety and worry can be very useful. Thinking that something bad may happen in the future if you don't take appropriate action motivates you to study for a test, learn your lines for a play, work on solutions to problems, and do your best when you perform. Anxiety's most important function is to prepare you for the possibility of danger in the future. When you are in an anxious state, you're already a little tense and alert, so it's easy to shift into the fight-or-flight response, which is your body's natural fear reaction to imminent danger or threat.

For example, when you're driving on a stormy day, you may feel a little anxious and tense. Rather than daydreaming or listening to the radio, you're likely to hold the steering wheel with both hands, sit up straight, and scan the road for possible threat. When you see a large tree falling just ahead of you, your emotion moves from anxious to fearful as your fight-or-flight response is triggered, and you respond instantly by braking and steering your car away from the danger.

Anxiety becomes a problem when it is triggered too frequently, is too intense, or you can't turn it off (Craske and Barlow 2006). If you are always anxious and worried, your body is always prepared for the possibility of danger in the future. While you won't go crazy from it, long-term anxiety and worry are likely to cause sleep problems, fatigue, irritability, and poor concentration, which can negatively impact your performance and productivity.

Anxiety can be triggered by anything perceived as potentially dangerous or threatening, such as the possibility of making a mistake, being rejected, missing a deadline, or not doing well on a test. The danger doesn't even have to be real, because simply thinking it might occur sometime in the future produces anxiety. People create unnecessary anxiety for themselves when they obsess about the danger of a possible future event as well as exaggerate the likelihood that it will actually occur. They wonder, *What if this terrible thing happens and I can't cope with it?* Then they think, *It would be a disaster!* Thoughts like these trigger anxiety.

Ana's Anxiety

It's Monday morning, and Ana is worried her children will be late for school and get into big trouble. She's also worried that she isn't prepared to give a five-minute speech at work today and will therefore blow it, even though she has been working on it for two weeks, and she's worried that her sick brother, at home with a cold, could get pneumonia.

Ana, like most chronically anxious people, does what she can to prevent bad things from happening. She overprepares for work because she is worried she will be criticized and perhaps even lose her job if she makes a mistake. She gets herself and her children to appointments early so as not to impolitely barge in late or miss something important. She checks things repeatedly, because she worries that if she didn't, disaster might result. Ironically, these *safety behaviors* perpetuate her anxiety because they prevent her from learning that it's highly unlikely anything catastrophic would happen if she didn't do these things, and that if there were a mishap, she probably could handle it.

So what if her kids were occasionally a few minutes late to school? She might get a call from the school, but the kids wouldn't fail or be kicked out. Checking on her sick brother many times a day may provide her with momentary reassurance, but it won't prevent pneumonia.

While worrying and engaging in safety behaviors, everyone becomes stressed. Ana goes to bed Sunday night worrying about her problems, and this makes her feel keyed up rather than sleepy. After tossing and turning in bed for an hour, she gets up to make her children's lunches rather than leaving this chore to them as she normally would. She does this because she thinks it might prevent her children from being late to school. She recalls the disapproving look on the school principal's face last week when the kids were late, and she feels a wave of fear as well as more tension in her shoulders.

She says to herself, *The principal must think I'm an incompetent mother. Maybe I'm not cut out to work and raise kids on my own.* Her stomach feels queasy. *What if they're not getting enough of my time? What if they start thinking it's okay to be late? What if they start turning their homework in late…maybe not do it at all? I can't handle all this and my job too!* She massages the pain that is spreading across her shoulders and takes an antacid to quell her upset stomach. *I'm so wired…if I don't get some sleep, I won't be functional tomorrow.* She returns to bed, sets her alarm to go off a half hour earlier than usual, and tosses and turns for another hour before falling asleep.

As you can see, worry, safety behaviors, and tension interact to escalate and maintain anxiety. This chapter is based on the work of Michelle Craske and David Barlow (2006), Steven Hayes (Hayes and Smith 2005), Melisa Robichaud and Michel Dugas (2015), and Mary Ellen Copeland (1998). It addresses the three components of anxiety that work together to maintain your anxiety and worry over time:

1. Your thoughts that tell you there is a possibility of danger or threat in the future

2. Your body, which becomes tense in response to this alert message

3. Your behaviors that are designed to check for danger and avoid it if possible

Symptom-Relief Effectiveness

The skills taught in this chapter will help you reduce your anxiety and worry and lessen the physical symptoms of tension associated with excessive worry, such as feeling restless, keyed up, or nervous, sleep disturbances, tiredness, difficulty concentrating, muscle tension, and irritability. These skills will also decrease the frequency of your spontaneous fear-provoking images of disaster and cut down on your safety behaviors.

Time to Master

You can learn and apply these skills within a few months. Move at a pace you are comfortable with as you work your way through the exercises in this chapter. Your success will depend on how much you practice these exercises.

Instructions

Relaxation Skills for General and Acute Tension Relief

Physical tension both contributes to and results from worry and anxiety. You can use the relaxation skills you've been learning in this book to begin to intervene in your cycle of anxiety and worry. If you haven't already mastered diaphragmatic breathing, turn to chapter 3 and begin with the first exercise under Breathing Basics to observe how you currently breathe. Then move on to diaphragmatic or abdominal breathing.

Next, turn to chapter 7 and learn the first three stages of applied relaxation. That is, practice progressive muscle relaxation, release-only relaxation, and cue-controlled relaxation. Your goal is to be able to relax in two or three minutes using cue-controlled relaxation techniques. As you practice this exercise, be sure to focus on the sensations of relaxation in your body, especially in your chest, abdomen, forehead, and shoulders.

To bring down your general level of arousal and tension associated with anxiety and worry, set aside time once or twice a day to relax for twenty minutes. Use this time to learn and practice diaphragmatic or abdominal breathing and the first three exercises in chapter 7. Keep a log of your level of relaxation at the beginning and end of each twenty-minute session, using the Record of General Tension from chapter 2 (visit http://www.newharbinger.com/43348 to download this resource).

Once you have successfully paired the word "relax" in the exercise Cue-Controlled Relaxation with the sensations of deep relaxation, start using cue-controlled relaxation whenever you feel your tension beginning to mount during the day.

Step Back and Observe Your Anxiety

It's hard to change something until you understand it. So to become more aware of the various components of your own anxiety, you will need to keep a daily record of your anxious thoughts, sensations of tension, and safety behaviors, so you can observe how they interact to cause your anxiety to escalate. According to Craske and Barlow (2006), you will become more detached and objective about your anxiety, worry, and tension when you regularly monitor and record your anxious experiences. You will also use this information to practice the techniques presented in this chapter and gain greater control over your anxiety and worry. You can also monitor your improvement, and pinpoint those areas in which you still need to work further, by continuing to fill out Anxious Episode Record forms.

Visit http://www.newharbinger.com/43348 to download the Anxious Episode Record, adapted from Craske and Barlow's (2006) "Worry Record," and use this record whenever you notice a dramatic increase in your anxiety level, catch yourself worrying, or feel symptoms of physical tension. Following the blank form is an example of Ana's Anxious Episode Record.

Anxious Episode Record

Date: _____ Length of episode: _____

Anxiety Severity Scale

Put an X at the point on this scale that best describes your maximum level of anxiety during this episode:

0	1	2	3	4	5	6	7	8	9	10
None		Mild			Moderate		Strong			Extreme

Triggering events:

_____

_____

_____

Worries:

_____

_____

_____

_____

Underline and/or fill in physical symptoms: muscle tension, sleep difficulties, difficulty concentrating, mind going blank, irritability, fatigue, restlessness, feeling keyed up or on edge. Other:

_____

_____

_____

Safety behaviors:

_____

_____

_____

Ana's Anxious Episode Record

Date: _____ 5/5 _____   Length of episode: _____ 5 hours _____

Anxiety Severity Scale

Put an X at the point on this scale that best describes your maximum level of anxiety during this episode.

0	1	2	3	4	5	6	7	8	9 ✘	10
None		Mild			Moderate		Strong			Extreme

Triggering events:

Five-minute presentation tomorrow at work, children late to school last week, brother sick

Worries:

I'm going to blow my presentation tomorrow and my boss will think I'm incompetent and fire me; my kids will be late to school and the principal will think that I'm an incompetent mother. What if my kids start being late about other things like homework? I couldn't handle that! What if my brother's cold turns into pneumonia? He could die! I wouldn't know what to do with such a terrible loss.

Underline and/or fill in physical symptoms: muscle tension, sleep difficulties, difficult concentrating, mind going blank, irritability, fatigue, restlessness, feeling keyed up or on edge. Other:

Upset stomach, pain in shoulders

Safety behaviors:

Make children's lunches and set alarm a half hour early to prevent their being late, overprepare for five-minute presentation, check on sick brother many times a day

---

As you use the following techniques to gain greater control over your anxiety and worry, you can continue to use the Anxious Episode Record to monitor your improvement and pinpoint areas where you need to work further.

Thought Defusion

Defusion is a treatment process developed by Stephen Hayes (Hayes and Smith 2005) and is part of a comprehensive psychotherapy called acceptance and commitment therapy (ACT). Defusion derives from the Buddhist practice of observing the mind—watching thoughts come and go rather than getting caught up in the content of your worries. Observing your mind, while labeling and releasing thoughts, can help you detach from catastrophic worries and take them much less seriously. You learn to see a thought as just that—a thought, one of about sixty thousand you'll have in a day. You can also learn to let thoughts pass and drift away, because they aren't real; they are merely a product of your mind. Your mind will always continue to pop out worry thoughts, but your relationship to them will be different. You'll be able to say to yourself, *There's a worry thought*, and let it go rather than dwell on it.

Mindful Focusing

Learning to defuse (decouple) from worry thoughts starts with *mindful focusing*, noticing your thoughts. Begin with your breath, putting attention on your diaphragm—the center and genesis of your breath. Say to yourself "in" on the in-breath and "out" on the out-breath.

Invariably, as you focus on your breath, thoughts will intrude. Every time they do, say "thought" to yourself, and return attention to your breath. No matter how carefully you observe your breath, thoughts inevitably show up. That's normal; you're doing nothing wrong. So the sequence is: breathe, notice a thought arising, label the thought, and return your focus to your breath.

Mindful focusing will help you learn to watch your mind, recognizing it as a veritable popcorn machine of thoughts, and give you some distance and separation from worry. Do this exercise for five minutes, twice a day.

Labeling Thoughts

Once you've learned to watch your mind via mindful focusing, it's time to start labeling upsetting thoughts as they show up in daily life—particularly your worries. You can do this in two ways. The first way is to say to yourself, "I'm having the thought that…" and then adding in whatever the thought is. For example, "I'm having the thought that I could get sick," or "I'm having the thought that I could lose my job," or "I'm having the thought that I'm going to play badly in front of my friends." Notice how prefacing each worry with "I'm having the thought that…" reminds you that this is a product of mind as opposed to actual fact. Labeling difficult thoughts in this way—whenever you notice them—is a discipline that can begin to liberate you from the tyranny of worry.

A second way to label thoughts is to remind yourself of what kind of thought it is. Anxiety-inducing thoughts about the future can be labeled *worry thoughts*. Or you could call them *C-thoughts*, where C stands for *catastrophic*. Now, every time you start worrying, identify it by saying "worry," or "C thought." The label reminds you that these are just thoughts. You can notice them without drowning in them.

Letting Go of Thoughts

Each time a worry thought shows up, let it go. You can schedule some time later to review your worries, if you want. You can even write down your worry thoughts in a notebook, so you won't forget them at your appointed worry time (a technique called *worry delay*). But at the moment the thought shows up, rather than dwelling on it, you can learn to let it go. One strategy for letting thoughts go is to use an image—like imagining the thought is on a billboard as you speed past it. Or seeing the thought drifting away like an untethered balloon. Or imagining the thought to be like a computer pop-up—suddenly appearing on your screen and then disappearing when you hit the close key.

You can also use physical movements to signal the letting-go process. One example is to take a deep breath and let go of the worry thought as you exhale. Imagine the thought being released with the out-breath. Another strategy is to drop the thought. Imagine you are holding the thought in your hand, palm up. Now rotate your hand so the palm faces down, imagining you are simultaneously letting the thought go. Do this gesture for every worry thought that arises.

Distancing from Worry Thoughts

One way to get emotional distance from distressing thoughts is to thank your mind for them:

Thank you, mind, for that worry thought.

Thank you, mind, for the thought I won't make my sales quota.

Thank you, mind, for the thought that I'll have an accident.

The mantra acknowledges that your mind is trying to protect you, while it also helps you not to get so involved in the thought. You don't have to understand or explore the thought—just thank your mind and let it go.

Another distancing strategy is simply to repeat the thought, over and over (up to sixty or seventy times) until it loses all meaning. This technique is called *Titchener's repetition*, after Edward Titchener, who discovered that words get stripped of meaning if they are repeated enough.

Still another approach to distancing from worry is to objectify the thought. Imagine that the thought has a color, a shape, a texture, or a certain size. For example, you could imagine that a worry thought is green and as big and round as a soccer ball. Now you can imagine just kicking it away. As an alternative, ask yourself how old the thought is—how many years have gone by since it first occurred to you? Imagine the thought as an old man with a cane, limping around a corner and out of sight.

Commit to Defusing Worry Thoughts

Defusion will help you change your relationship to worry—if you use it. Right now, commit to using one or more defusion strategies each time you notice a worry thought. It might be as simple as saying to yourself *There's a worry thought* and visualizing it drifting away like a leaf down a stream. Or you could just take a deep breath at the first sign of worry and imagine the thought blowing away as you exhale. Or you could notice a worry, write it down to think about later (worry delay), and thank your mind for another worry thought.

The keys to successful defusion and distancing from worry are:

1. Notice worry thoughts as soon as possible. At the moment you become aware of worrying, you have a choice: to keep worrying or to label and let go of the thought.

2. Use your defusion strategies every time a worry thought shows up. Make it a habit by committing yourself to responding to worry with some form of distancing or letting go.

3. Diversify your defusion strategies. Keep mixing them up so you try something new every so often.

4. Deal with sticky worry thoughts aggressively. Use techniques like the old man visualization or Titchener's repetition to make fun of the thought or help it lose meaning.

Change Your Safety Behaviors

We're all hardwired to protect ourselves from dangerous situations. When we experience threat, we'll act quickly and go to great lengths to feel safe. If you were in an unlit parking garage and you heard footsteps behind you, it's likely that you'd move more quickly to get to the safety of your car. In addition to seeking safety in response to a physically threatening situation, you may find yourself seeking safety to alleviate the anxiety you experience when you worry about something. *Safety behaviors* are chosen actions that are carried out to protect you from the emotion of fear, and the catastrophes you worry about. Safety behaviors are compelling because they provide immediate benefits in that they reduce the *feeling* of danger in the short term.

The Problem with Safety Behaviors

One of the main problems with using safety behaviors is that you never get to find out whether your feared situation can hurt you. In fact, avoiding what you fear will increase anxiety over time. For example, suppose you worry a lot about making decisions, trying to think ahead to see all the possible bad outcomes. The worry is designed to help you get rid of uncertainty, but it doesn't—each projected bad outcome only increases your sense of uncertainty and threat. Your anxiety intensifies. This is where you start turning to safety behaviors. Perhaps you procrastinate, or you make a decision while continually seeking reassurance and advice. The ultimate outcome of these safety behaviors is that you never learn to tolerate uncertainty or trust your own judgment. Every decision continues to make you anxious.

The following sequence shows how safety behaviors maintain—and often worsen—anxiety.

Specific threat: something that creates uncertainty about safety

↓

Worry: thinking about catastrophic things that could happen in hopes of reducing uncertainty (threat)

↓

Anxiety/fear increases the longer you worry.

↓

Safety behaviors help you avoid threat or somehow reduce it.

↓

Anxiety temporarily decreases.

↓

No learning takes place that the threat can't hurt you; you don't learn to tolerate uncertainty.

↓

Specific threat reappears.

↓

Sequence repeats.

Types of Safety Behaviors

So safety behaviors provide temporary relief but keep you from learning that most of the situations you worry about won't end in catastrophe. Now that you understand the purpose of—and problem with—safety behaviors, let's look at what types of safety behaviors you might engage in.

Excessive Reassurance Seeking

If this is one of your safety behaviors, you seek reassurance from others when you are worrying about a decision. This might include making a big decision, like the purchase of a car, or a smaller decision, like what to have for dinner. While it's normal to ask others for their opinions, *excessive reassurance seeking* is a safety behavior, because you are asking multiple times in order to counteract the anxiety that your worry generates.

Distraction

When facing a feared experience, you might behave in ways that are meant to distract you. This could include daydreaming, compulsive TV watching or Internet use, counting, tapping, planning, and so on.

Procrastination

Procrastination is a safety behavior that falls under the broader category of avoidance. With procrastination, you're putting off a feared experience as a way to delay worrying about something or to minimize your sense of threat or risk.

Checking and Double-Checking

With this safety behavior you might double-check that you turned off the stove before you leave your home, or you may check on loved ones several times a day to make sure they are safe. This is your attempt to feel less anxious when faced with uncertainty.

Avoidance

With avoidance, you reduce your anxiety by getting away from a situation that seems uncertain and threatening. You might avoid getting your annual checkup because you don't know what the doctor is going to tell you. You might avoid tasks or challenges where you worry about failure.

Overpreparation

The activities around this safety behavior are designed to increase your certainty about situations that are ambiguous or unpredictable. Maybe you've heard the expression, "I'm anxious about anything I can't Google." You will seek out as much information and prepare yourself as much as possible to decrease the level of uncertainty when you face a worry-provoking challenge.

Perfectionism

The goal of this safety behavior is to do everything flawlessly to eliminate uncertainty and mistakes. This means not delegating tasks to others, so that you can make sure the tasks get done the way you want. It can also mean overworking to avoid the possibility of errors.

Drugs/Alcohol/Anxiety Medications

Trying to mute anxiety with drugs or alcohol is a safety behavior. So is keeping anxiety medications with you as a precaution, just in case you have an anxiety attack.

Generalized Anxiety Disorder (Worry) and Safety Behaviors

Generalized anxiety disorder (GAD) and worry are maintained by the use of safety behaviors. As you gradually eliminate safety behaviors, you'll become more tolerant of uncertainty, and your anxiety (fear of uncertainty) will gradually diminish. Therefore, discontinuing safety behaviors is absolutely essential to overcoming worry and GAD.

The first step in overcoming worry is to develop a Worry Inventory. The inventory focuses on situations that trigger worry, the specific worry generated by that situation, and the safety behavior you use to cope with the worry-induced anxiety.

To get started on the Worry Inventory, think about recent worries and the situations that induced them. In column 1, describe the situation; in column 2, list your worry (a feared catastrophic outcome); in column 3, name your coping strategy to minimize anxiety for that particular situation or worry.

Worry Inventory

Situation	Worry	Safety Behavior

Stephan, who struggled with a harsh *worry voice*, completed his worry inventory as follows:

Stephan's Worry Inventory

Situation	Worry	Safety Behavior
Stomach pain/gas	Fear doctors are wrong—it's serious.	Online medical research
Work deadline	What if I miss it? Getting fired/humiliated.	Constantly listing things to be done; checking list; reassurance seeking with colleagues
Stock market goes down	Will it crash? Lose everything.	Constantly check DOW and S&P; call broker for reassurance
Buying a new car: Buick	It'll be a lemon. I won't like it.	Recheck Consumer Reports. Procrastinate; frequent test drives (checking).
Recent mass shooting + going to concert	I'll be killed. The concert will be targeted.	Reassurance seeking with friends; checking news stories about terrorist activities
Boss asking for a meeting	I'll be reprimanded or fired.	Reassurance seeking with colleagues
High heart rate at gym	Do I have heart disease? Coming heart attack?	Online medical research; constantly checking pulse
Condo needing new roof and paint	Cost will force me to sell my home/ financial trouble.	Checking condo prices; check DOW & S&P

Notice that Stephan used multiple safety behaviors, even at times for the same worry, and the particular safety behaviors were usually associated with a specific type of worries (health worries, job worries, financial worries, and so on). It was crucial for Stephan to realize that his safety behaviors were maintaining his worry and that they kept him intolerant of uncertainty. If he was going to reduce worry and anxiety in his life, he would have to discontinue his safety behaviors.

Discontinuing Worry-Driven Safety Behaviors

Discontinuing worry-based safety behaviors can be accomplished either cold turkey or with a gradual hierarchy. The Safety Behavior Planning Worksheet is where you can develop a discontinuation plan for each worry-based safety behavior. In the first column, fill in your safety behavior (organized by type), and in the second column, enter your corresponding discontinuation plan. The behavioral test in the third column will be covered in the next section. You don't need to deal with that now.

Safety Behavior Planning Worksheet

Safety Behavior	Plan	Behavioral Test

Stephan transferred the list of his safety behaviors from his Worry Inventory to a Safety Behavior Planning Worksheet. Here's how he filled it out:

Stephan's Safety Behavior Planning Worksheet

Safety Behavior	Plan	Behavioral Test
Checking:		
Online medical research	Discontinue.	
DOW and S&P	Decrease from 2x to 1x every other day, then discontinue.	
Consumer Reports	Discontinue.	
Condo prices	Check once, then discontinue.	
Driving new cars	Drive each model once, for a total of five models, then discontinue.	
Physical symptoms (pulse)	Check 2x per day, then 1x per day, then discontinue.	
Disaster news stories; news in general	Discontinue.	
To-do list making and checking	Add items 1x daily; check 1x daily only.	
Reassurance seeking from broker, friends, colleagues	Quarterly consult only with broker; stop discussing fears with friends or colleagues.	
Procrastinating	Set date for decision now.	

Behavioral Testing

There's an additional step you can take to overcome safety behaviors. This process—*behavioral testing*—gives you an opportunity to see if safety behaviors really keep you safe. It allows you to test the belief that failing to do safety behaviors, like checking or reassurance seeking, will result in catastrophe.

Here's how it works. Identify a particular type of safety behavior that you often rely on—one that shows up in your Safety Behavior Planning Worksheet. Now you can set up experiments to discontinue this behavior across several contexts or situations. For example, Stephan might experiment with stopping his checking behavior with physical symptoms, disaster news, and stock market reports. Then for each experiment, he'd predict what would likely happen—a feared outcome. After stopping the safety behavior, Stephan would record what actually happened to complete the experiment.

Stephan's behavioral testing sequence looked like this:

Example 1:

Test: *Discontinue checking my pulse.*

Prediction: *I'll have heart trouble and not know it. When I see the doctor next week, he'll tell me I had a "silent heart attack."*

Outcome: *The doctor said my heart was fine.*

Example 2:

Test: *Discontinue checking stocks.*

Prediction: *The market will plunge in the next week and I won't know it—too late to sell.*

Outcome: *The market actually went up.*

Example 3:

Test: *Checking to-do list one time daily.*

Prediction: *I'll forget to do something vital and will make a gross screwup at work.*

Outcome: *Two weeks into this test, I haven't forgotten anything except calling an old client—no big deal.*

As he completed each test, Stephan recorded his predictions and outcomes in the third column of his Safety Behavior Planning Worksheet. Stephan did additional tests of his checking safety behavior in some other situations that were not on his worksheet:

- *Don't check with my girlfriend to see if she's still available for our plans.*

- *Don't check with my mother about her health—let her tell me if something's wrong.*

- *Stop checking to see if my glands are swollen.*

With behavioral testing, Stephan learned that his feared outcomes didn't happen, and over time he was able to discontinue his safety behaviors.

Turn Worry into Problem Solving

In this chapter, so far you've learned how to deal more realistically with exaggerated worries. But what can you do to keep your worry from getting out of hand when you have a life crisis or genuine problem? There are three practical steps you can take to minimize your worry and anxiety:

1. Clearly define the problem.

2. Use brainstorming to find solutions.

3. Make a contract with yourself to follow through on your solutions.

The following step-by-step model for turning worry into problem solving was adapted from the *Worry Control Workbook* by Mary Ellen Copeland (1998). Each step is followed by an example of how a young entrepreneur used this problem-solving process to deal with worries about starting her business. Following this model is a blank Problem-Solving Worksheet for you to use with this technique.

1. Write down one situation that is really worrying you. Be specific about what the problem is. Example: *I really want to start a business of my own, but my financial resources are very limited. I'm worried that I don't know enough to avoid the pitfalls, and I'll end up losing everything.*

2. Brainstorm for solutions. Make a list of possible things you can do to improve or correct the situation.

- *Talk to other entrepreneurs about their experiences in starting their businesses.*

- *Research organizations that support entrepreneurial efforts and people.*

- *Research the possibility of acquiring a small-business loan or other capital available for small start-up businesses.*

- *Join a couple of small-business and entrepreneurial organizations.*

- *Find investors among friends and family.*

- *Start the business out of my home to save overhead and protect me financially.*

- *Work an extra job for a couple of years to earn more money.*

- *Stay at current job while starting my own company part time.*

3. Evaluate each idea. Which ideas are not possible? Put an X next to those. Which ones would be difficult to implement? Put a question mark next to those. Which ideas could you implement right now? Put a Y next to those.

Talk to other entrepreneurs about their experiences starting their businesses.	Y
Research organizations that support entrepreneurial efforts and people.	Y
Research the possibility of acquiring a small-business loan or other capital available for small start-up businesses.	Y
Join a couple of small-business and entrepreneurial organizations.	?
Find investors among family and friends.	Y
Start the business out of my own home to save overhead.	?
Work an extra job for a couple of years to earn more money.	X
Stay at current job while starting the company part time.	X

4. Set specific dates. Make a contract with yourself to do all the things that you've marked with a Y.

    By April 1, I will talk to other entrepreneurs about their experiences in starting their businesses.

    By April 15, I will research organizations that support entrepreneurial efforts and people.

    By May 1, I'll have canvassed family and friends for possible investors.

    By May 15, I will research the possibility of acquiring a small-business loan or other capital available for small start-up businesses.

5. When you have completed all of the items marked with a Y, go on to the more difficult things marked with a question mark. Make a contract with yourself to do those as well.

    By June 15, I will join a couple of small-business and entrepreneurial organizations.

    By July 1, I'll decide whether I should clear out a back bedroom to create a home-based business office.

6. Now, maybe some of the items marked with an X don't look so hard. If there are any that you think you could manage, make a contract with yourself to take that action: *By August 15, if other options have not worked out, I will start my company part time while continuing to work full time at my job.*

Use the blank Problem-Solving Worksheet to apply this same problem-solving technique to one of your worries. Visit http://www.newharbinger.com/43348 to download this worksheet for further use.

Problem-Solving Worksheet

Choose a situation that is really worrying you, and apply this problem-solving technique:

1. Write down the situation that is really worrying you.

   _____

   _____

   _____

2. Brainstorm for solutions. Make a list of possible things you can do to improve or correct the situation.

   _____

   _____

   _____

   _____

3. Evaluate each idea. Which ones are not possible? Put an X next to those. Which ones would be difficult to implement? Put a question mark next to those. Which ones could you do right now? Put a Y next to those.

4. Set specific dates. Make a contract with yourself to do all the Y items.

- By _____ (date), I will _____.

- By _____ (date), I will _____.

- By _____ (date), I will _____.

- By _____ (date), I will _____.

5. When you have completed the Y items, go on to the more difficult items. Make a contract with yourself to do those as well.

- By _____ (date), I will _____.

- By _____ (date), I will _____.

- By _____ (date), I will _____.

- By _____ (date), I will _____.

6. Now, maybe some of the X items don't look so hard. If there are any that you think you could manage, make a contract with yourself to take that action.

- By _____ (date), I will _____.

- By _____ (date), I will _____.

- By _____ (date), I will _____.

- By _____ (date), I will _____.

Note that three other chapters in this workbook can help you deal with life problems. Chapter 16 helps with goal setting and time management, chapter 17 offers assertiveness training, and chapter 18 focuses on work-stress management.

Final Thoughts

Facing your worry and anxiety will become progressively easier as you regularly practice the skills presented in this chapter. Consider these goals for yourself. Each time you choose to use your relaxation skills, you will feel less tense. Each time you successfully defuse from worry thoughts, you will experience more peace of mind. Each time you tackle situations that you are worried about—and don't experience the negative consequences that you feared—you will become a little more self-confident and resilient. Each time you focus on problem solving, you will become more aware of the many resources you have to accomplish your goals. Just be patient with yourself as you practice these skills, because it takes a while to overcome old habits of thinking and behaving and to develop new ones.

Further Reading

Barlow, D. H. 2001. *Anxiety and Its Disorders. The Nature and Treatment of Anxiety and Panic.* 2nd ed. New York: Guilford Press.

Brown, T. A., R. M. Hertz, and D. H. Barlow. 1992. "New Developments in Cognitive-Behavioral Treatment of Anxiety Disorders." In *American Psychiatric Press Review of Psychiatry*, vol. 2, edited by A. Tasman. Washington, DC: American Psychiatric Press. Out of print.

Copeland, M. E. 1998. *Worry Control Workbook.* Oakland, CA: New Harbinger Publications. Out of print.

Craske, M. G., and D. H. Barlow. 2006. *Mastery of Your Anxiety and Worry.* 2nd ed. New York: Oxford University Press.

Hayes, S. C., and S. Smith. 2005. *Get Out of Your Mind and Into Your Life.* Oakland, CA: New Harbinger Publications.

McKay, M., M. Davis, and P. Fanning. 2011. *Thoughts and Feelings: Taking Control of Your Moods and Your Life.* 4th ed. Oakland, CA: New Harbinger Publications.

O'Leary, T. A., T. A. Brown, and D. H. Barlow. 1992. "The Efficacy of Worry Control Treatment in Generalized Anxiety Disorder: A Multiple Baseline Analysis." Paper presented at the annual meeting of the Association for Advancement of Behavior Therapy, Boston.

Robichaud, M., and M. J. Dugas. 2015. *The Generalized Anxiety Disorder Workbook.* Oakland, CA: New Harbinger Publications.

White, J. 1999. *Overcoming Generalized Anxiety Disorder. Therapist Protocol.* Oakland, CA: New Harbinger Publications.

CHAPTER 14

Facing Fear and Avoidance

In this chapter you will learn to:

■ Face fear-provoking situations that you currently avoid or endure with considerable discomfort

■ Disprove catastrophic beliefs that fuel your fear and anxiety and keep you from doing things you value

■ Significantly lower your fear and anxiety

Background

Avoidance is a great way to escape danger and reduce fear and anxiety quickly, but it needlessly restricts a person's life when the feared experience isn't a real theat. Phobias can develop when something like a spider becomes linked to fearful thoughts, feelings, and sensations as a result of a frightening experience; for instance, a playmate drops a harmless spider down a little girl's shirt and shouts, "Spider!" Phobias can also be learned by observing others: a child sees her terrified babysitter repeatedly jump on top of a chair, screaming, whenever she sees a daddy longlegs on the floor. Due to this *classical conditioning*, once the child pairs a previously neutral stimulus with danger, she responds with fear whenever she encounters a spider. She becomes anxious and worried when she thinks about spiders. As much as possible, she organizes her life to avoid what she believes will harm her.

A person with a phobia can become locked in an endless loop of fear and avoidance that prevents new, more adaptive learning. While most spiders aren't dangerous, people who live in areas with poisonous spiders learn to deal with them without getting hurt. But the little girl who avoids what she believes is dangerous cuts herself off from opportunities to learn more effective ways to respond to spiders. She also doesn't learn that she can tolerate some distress when around spiders rather than run away. Instead, she inflates their danger in her mind and underestimates her ability to cope with them. So she becomes stuck with her phobia, and her world becomes a little smaller as she unconsciously crosses off life choices that might include a spider. Only when she realizes that her fear and avoidance cause her to miss out on aspects of her life that she values does she become motivated to face her fear and stop avoiding.

Until recently, the gold standard for treating fearful avoidance has been exposure therapy based on a *habituation* model (McKay, Skeen, and Fanning 2017). Clients would be exposed repeatedly to a fear-provoking situation, such as a spider, in the absence of an adverse outcome, until they were no longer afraid. Over the years exposure therapy has often been combined with various cognitive behavioral strategies to help clients rationally challenge their catastrophic beliefs about their phobias, as well as with coping statements and relaxation techniques to mitigate their fear and arousal. For example, Wolpe's (1958) *systematic desensitization* helped clients rid themselves of their fear and avoidance by teaching them relaxation techniques and then taking them through a hierarchical list of exposure exercises involving their least to most feared situations in the absence of negative outcomes. They would visualize a distressing situation on their hierarchy until it no longer evoked fearful arousal. Once habituated, they would move on to the next item on their hierarchy and repeat the process. Treatment was considered successful when they could experience all the items on their hierarchy with little or no fear or arousal. In the 1980s, Edna Foa (Foa and Kozak 1986) extended the habituation model by eliminating relaxation and using prolonged *in vivo* exposures.

Many people have overcome their fear and avoidance using exposure therapy based on the habituation model. However, it can be time-consuming, and it does not work for everybody. Long-term follow-up tests indicate that some clients relapsed after successfully completing exposure programs. These studies have shown that the reduction of fear within exposure sessions and at the completion of exposure treatment doesn't guarantee that the fear won't reemerge at some point after the end of treatment (Craske et al. 2008). This has led cognitive behavioral therapists to look for a more efficient and more effective treatment for fearful avoidance.

Craske and her associates (2014) developed a faster, more effective exposure program based on an *inhibitory learning model*. This program shifts away from a goal of reducing fear and physical arousal. Instead, it facilitates new learning that contradicts and overrides (inhibits) the unhelpful fear-based old learning.

Here is how it works. The client asks himself two questions: *What is the worst possible outcome that could happen if I experience the situation that I have been avoiding?* and *How likely do I feel that this expectation will occur?* He then designs exposure exercises to test his catastrophic expectation. At the conclusion of each exposure practice, he compares his expectation of a dreadful outcome with what actually takes place. The greater the difference between his catastrophic expectation of what will happen and what actually occurs, the greater his surprise and the greater the opportunity will be to learn something new and more adaptive. People need to have that their beliefs about danger disconfirmed before they change. It is not enough to dispute these beliefs rationally (McKay, Skeen, and Fanning 2017).

It is important to preserve the power of surprise and new learning that comes with experiencing the discrepancy between the client's fearful expectation of outcome and what actually occurs during an exposure exercise. Craske and associates (2014) advise saving relaxation exercises and cognitive interventions that emphasize logic and facts (for example, rational emotive therapy) for after the exposure exercise when the client contemplates the meaning of what actually happened versus his fearful expectation.

This exposure program takes determination. Some people courageously face their feared situation almost immediately following this program. When they do, they are pleasantly surprised to learn that their fearful expectations are not true, and their fear and avoidance subsides. Others need to approach these fearful situations at their own pace, moving more gradually from less challenging to more challenging exposure sessions. While this takes longer, they are rewarded for their courage and hard work. If facing their fearful situation alone seems too scary, they also have the option to do this exposure program with the support of a friend or a therapist.

Symptom-Relief Effectiveness

Studies show that compared to other forms of cognitive behavioral therapy, exposure therapy, based on the concept of inhibitory learning, works the fastest to correct erroneous beliefs related to a feared situation, overcome avoidant behavior, and reduce anxiety and physiological arousal. And these results are long lasting (Craske et al. 2014; McKay, Skeen, and Fanning 2017).

Time to Master

It may take an hour or two to complete the Fear and Avoidance Assessment Form. The exposure program then consists of three steps: planning an exposure session, experiencing the exposure session, and debriefing the exposure session during which new learning is consolidated. These three steps are repeated until your fear and avoidance diminish to a level where you are convinced that your fearful expectation is highly unlikely to occur and you can confidently experience the situation you previously avoided or tolerated with distress. The length of time needed to complete this exposure program will vary from a few days to several months.

Instructions

Assess the Impact of Fearful Avoidance in Your Life

This program takes motivation. Sometimes a major life change gives a person a nudge. Such was the case for Cindy, a new mother with a phobia of elevators. She soon found it exhausting to carry her fast-growing baby and all his baby paraphernalia up and down the four flights of her apartment building. She used this program to overcome her fear of elevators and saved herself a lot of time and energy by taking her apartment building's lift.

If you are wondering if this program is for you, this assessment exercise will help you look at the consequences to your life of avoiding situations you fear or enduring these situations with distress. Fill out the blank Fear and Avoidance Assessment Form after reading the instructions in the following example.

Helena's Fear and Avoidance Assessment Form

1. What do you avoid or endure with distress? Pick one of your feared situations for this exercise. If you fear multiple situations, use a blank Fear and Avoidance Assessment Form for each feared situation.

    I fear and avoid, as much as I possibly can, spiders, public speaking, flying, and riding in elevators. I will work on public speaking first.

2. What do you believe is the worst outcome that you expect could happen if you faced your fear situation? The emphasis here is what you believe would happen, not what others (even the experts) tell you is the rational thing that could happen.

    I'll be so nervous speaking in front of my audience that my mind will go blank, and I won't be able to speak or I'll stumble over my words. I worry that the audience will think I'm a complete idiot and they'll get up and walk out or they'll laugh at me and then ignore me. If my boss is in the audience, it will mean my job!

3. What are examples of situations you avoid or endure with distress because of this fearful expectation? Take time to think about this question across various areas of your life: for example, friendship, family, work, education, health/self-care, pleasure/recreation, life goals, service to others, and romantic relationships (McKay, Skeen, and Fanning 2017).

    At work, I avoid whenever possible giving status reports to my team and presentations to management or at conventions. At family gatherings and when I'm with a group of my friends, I avoid speaking to the whole group at once. In classes, at my service club, and at my apartment association meetings, I never ask questions or share my opinion unless called upon to do so.

4. In addition to avoiding, what are the other ways you minimize your fear for each of these examples? Examples of these safety behaviors include procrastinating, distraction, blocking, seeking reassurance from others, list making, checking and rechecking, postponing, overpreparing, perfectionism, and using drugs or alcohol (McKay, Skeen, and Fanning 2017).

    If I have to address a group at work, I first try to get a lot of reassurance about what I plan to say. I postpone my talk as long as possible. If I must give a speech, I read it as fast as I can, never making eye contact with anyone. In short, I block out the audience. When I'm at family functions or out with a group of my friends, I use alcohol to calm my nerves. At apartment meetings or a class, I always sit quietly in the back. If called upon, I give short answers or say "I don't know."

Fill in your answers to the following three questions on the chart that follows.

5. What would you like to do, experience, or accomplish if you didn't have this fearful expectation? This is a key question, since you are much more likely to tolerate some distress in order to do something that you value highly.

6. On a scale of 1 to 5, with 1 meaning "not at all" and 5 meaning "extremely," how much do you value each these experiences?

7. On a scale of 1 to 100, how distressing do you feel it will be to experience each of these feared situations, with 1 being "not at all" and 100 being "extremely distressing"?

5. Things you would like to do, experience, or accomplish	6. Value	7. Distress level
Present my idea for a new game to my work team.	5	80
Give a project update to management and make eye contact.	5	95
Demonstrate a new game at a convention and answer questions.	5	100
Give a toast at my best friend's wedding.	5	90
Ask questions and express my opinion at my service club.	3	60
Speak up at my apartment condo association meeting.	4	70
Ask and answer questions in class.	4	65
Tell a long story or joke to a group of my friends at lunch.	5	60
Express a contradictory opinion at a big family dinner.	5	65

8. In reviewing your answers to these questions, what have you learned?

I've always known I've had a problem with public speaking, but this exercise makes it painfully clear to me that if I want to progress in my career, I need to overcome my fear of speaking in groups. I also would like to be able to speak up in groups I'm part of outside of work. I'm sick and tired of worrying about freezing up when I speak to groups and worrying about people judging me as incompetent or stupid and rejecting me. I have a lot of good ideas, and I want to express them at work as well as in my personal life.

9. Are you willing to use this exposure program to stop avoiding and face your fear as you test your catastrophic expectations?

I'm willing to face my fear and do exposure work to challenge my nightmare expectations about speaking to groups.

Now fill out the blank form to assess the impact of fear and avoidance in your own life. You can also visit http://www.newharbinger.com/43348 to download this form.

Fear and Avoidance Assessment Form

1. What do you avoid or endure with distress?

   _____

   _____

2. What do you believe is the worst outcome that you expect could happen if you faced your fear situation?

   _____

   _____

   _____

   _____

3. What are examples of situations you avoid or endure with distress because of this fearful expectation?

   _____

   _____

   _____

   _____

4. What are examples of what you do to minimize your fear?

_____

_____

_____

_____

Fill in your answers to the following three questions on the chart that follows.

5. What would you like to do, experience, or accomplish if you didn't have this fearful expectation?

6. On a scale of 1 to 5, with 1 meaning "not at all" and 5 meaning "extremely," how much do you value each of these experiences?

7. On a scale of 1 to 100, how distressing do you feel it will be to experience your feared situations, with 1 being "not at all" and 100 being "extremely distressing"?

5. Things you would like to do, experience or accomplish	6. Value	7. Distress level

8. In reviewing you answers to these questions, what have you learned?

_____

_____

_____

_____

9. Are you willing to use this exposure program to stop avoiding and face your fear as you test your catastrophic expectations?

_____

_____

Planning Your First Exposure Exercise

By completing the Fear and Avoidance Assessment Form, you have already done most of the background work needed to plan and do your first exposure session. Read the following instructions with the example of how Helena took these steps. Then fill out your Exposure Exercise Planning Form, do your first exposure exercise, and complete your Exposure Exercise Debriefing Form.

1. For your first exposure exercise, review your answers to questions 5 through 7 on your Fear and Avoidance Assessment Form and pick an example of a feared situation that you value (a 4 or 5 on a 5-point scale) and that has one of the lowest distress ratings, ideally between 60 and 70 on a 100-point scale.

2. Identify the safety behaviors that you would usually use in this feared situation.

3. What is your catastrophic expectation of a negative outcome that could happen when you do your exposure exercise in this feared situation? Write a brief description of what you most worry could happen, full of observable behavior and events that you can use as evidence to confirm or disconfirm your catastrophic expectation. Don't predict that you'll feel afraid. Only predict the actual events that could happen. This will get easier as you practice.

Here are three examples to get you started. A shy man writes, "When I introduce myself to an attractive woman I don't know at Don's party, I will be so nervous that I will have trouble getting my words out. She will frown, back away, and make an excuse to get away from me as soon as possible." A man with a fear of heights writes: "When I am hiking up a mountain in the Sierras with my friends, I will look around at the view and become dizzy, lose my balance, and tumble to my death." A young woman with a fear of dogs writes: "While I'm jogging in the park, a big dog will attack me, biting me multiple times, causing me to have to go to the emergency room to stop the bleeding and have my wounds sutured."

4. On a scale of 1 to 100, how strongly do you believe that your catastrophic expectation will occur when you do your exposure exercise? Base your answer on your feelings, not logic and facts.

5. Plan your exposure exercise. Make a brief outline of what you want to do, experience, and/ or accomplish in your exposure session to disprove your expectation of a negative outcome when you face your fear situation. Be specific. What exactly are you going to do? What safety behaviors are you willing to forego? How much time do you need in your feared situation to test your catastrophic expectation? If distance is an issue, how near to your feared situation do you need to be? Think like a scientist. How will you need to set up the experiment (exposure exercise) to best test your hypothesis (catastrophic prediction)?

Remember that the bigger the discrepancy between your catastrophic expectation of what could happen when you expose yourself to your feared situation and what actually happens, the greater your new adaptive learning. So, dropping all of your safety behaviors at once will give you the biggest surprise when your catastrophic expectation doesn't happen. But if you think that this would be too overwhelming, you can eliminate one safety behavior at a time over several progressively more challenging exposure exercises. If being in the same room with your feared situation is something you are not ready to do, stand outside or begin with imagery, a written description, photos, or videos before attempting the real thing in progressively more challenging exposure sessions.

Decide when your exposure exercise will end. Stay in the exposure, no matter how anxious or tense you feel, until the time is up. An hour is a good length of time. But if an hour seems too long for an exposure exercise, cut the exercise into two half-hour sessions. For example, a woman with a fear of heights planned to stand by the balcony railing of a friend's apartment and look down at the garden six floors below for two thirty-minute periods, regardless of her level of fear or physical arousal. Another option is to set a behavioral goal. For example, a man with a fear of freeway driving planned to get on the freeway near his house and get off at the third exit, then drive around the block to get back on the freeway to drive home. If you are doing your exposure exercise and realize that your catastrophic expectation is not going to happen and your fear level has come down dramatically to about 15 or less, you can stop and do your debriefing.

Experience Your Exposure Exercise

Once you have written out your plan, go do your exposure exercise. As you experience your exposure session, pay attention to the details of what you and others are doing, how you're feeling, and what happens. It's natural to feel fearful. Accept your emotions and physical sensations. Notice their ebb and flow as you carry out your plan. Continue a given exposure session until either you are convinced that your catastrophic expectation is not going to happen or you have completed your specific behavioral or time goal.

Debriefing After Exposure

As soon as you have completed your exposure exercise, take time to summarize your experience and think about what you have learned by filling out the Exposure Exercise Debriefing Form.

For example, Helena did the three steps of exposure practice: planning her exposure exercise, doing the actual exposure, and debriefing. She began by going over her answers to questions 5 to 7 on the Fear and Avoidance Assessment Form. She chose an example of a feared situation that was important to her but not too distressing for her first exposure exercise.

Helena's Exposure Exercise Planning Form

Choose a feared situation you avoid or endure with distress:

Asking and answering questions in class.

Value (1–5): 4   Distress level (1–100): 65

Safety behaviors:

I sit in the back of the classroom, don't make eye contact, and say nothing unless spoken to. If I'm directly asked a question, my answer is as brief as possible or I say, "I don't know."

Catastrophic expectation of outcome:

If I volunteer to answer questions or if I ask questions, I'm afraid I will get so anxious that I will stumble over my words, so what I say will sound like nonsense and my classmates and teacher will laugh at me and say something mocking or critical.

Likelihood of your catastrophic expectation of outcome occurring: *65 percent*

Your exposure exercise plan:

At my next class, I will sit up front, look at the teacher, and answer in detail at least one question and ask at least one question. Even if I'm very anxious, I will speak up and finish my intended answer or question.

Helena followed through on her exposure exercise plan and right after class filled out her Exposure Exercise Debriefing Form.

Helena's Exposure Exercise Debriefing Form

Did what you were most worried about happen? No (X) Yes ( )

How do you know? List specific evidence telling you that your feared outcome did or didn't occur.

While I was nervous, I sat up front and looked the teacher in the eye. The first time I answered a question, I felt like my pounding heart was in my throat, which made talking difficult. I did stumble over my words once, but I managed to make sense and I answered correctly and in detail. I answered a second question, still nervous, but without stumbling. I also asked a question that I had been curious about for weeks. Everyone listened politely and nobody laughed at me.

What did you learn from doing this exposure exercise?

Even though I was scared and my heart pounded, I could make myself understood when I spoke. Nobody seems to judge me and reject me for being nervous when I speak. It was easier than I thought it would be going into it, but I need to keep answering and asking questions in future class meetings to become more confident doing this.

How likely (percent probability) do you feel your catastrophic expectation will occur the next time you are in this feared situation? *25 percent*

On a scale of 1 to 100, how intense was your distress about this feared situation before and after the exposure exercise?

Before: *65*   After: *30*

What do you need to learn now?

While my fear of being judged and rejected when I ask and answer questions in class has diminished, I want to get more practice doing this in class and in other situations. I see now how to set up similar exposure exercises at my service club, at family dinners, and when I'm out socializing with a group of my friends.

Helena practiced speaking up at her service club and in social situations with family and friends. Then she turned to the pressing matter of giving presentations at work. She filled out another Exposure Exercise Planning Form:

Helena's Exposure Exercise Planning Form

Choose a feared situation you avoid or endure with distress:

Giving a presentation about my new idea for a game to my team.

Value (1–5): 5   Distress level (1–100): 85

Safety behaviors:

Read my presentation word for word and fast, make no eye contact, and block out my audience.

Catastrophic expectation of outcome:

When I give an overview of my idea for a new game to my team next week, I will lose my concentration, start stammering, and won't be able to explain even the basics of its design. As a result, they'll think it is a stupid idea and ask a lot of critical questions.

Likelihood of your catastrophic expectation of outcome occurring: *80 percent*

Your exposure exercise plan:

I will give a presentation of my new game idea to my team at our regular team meeting in which I will cover the basics of its design. I won't write out a speech; I will have a note card with a short list of points I want to cover. I won't look at it if I don't need to. I will make eye contact with everyone in the audience and speak slowly. At the conclusion of my presentation, I will answer questions and ask for suggestions on how to improve the design.

Helena went ahead and carried out her exposure exercise at her next team meeting. She filled out her Exposure Exercise Debriefing Form shortly after the meeting.

Helena's Exposure Exercise Debriefing Form

Did what you were most worried about happen? No (X) Yes ( )

How do you know? List specific evidence telling you that your feared outcome did or didn't occur.

In spite of my pounding heart, dry mouth, sweaty armpits, and tripping a bit over my words at the beginning, I was able to explain my new game idea to my team. I looked only briefly at my notes, and I did make eye contact. I noticed that my body calmed down as my presentation went on. Rather than their rejecting my new game idea out of hand, we ended up having a lively exchange about its merits and ways it could be made even better. We agreed to discuss it in more depth at our next meeting. I was blown away!

What did you learn from doing this exposure exercise?

I learned that I could present a new idea for a game to my team in spite of my fear of criticism and my physical sensations of fear. I can use the feedback that I received to strengthen my game design by our next team meeting. I learned that at least with my peers, being afraid doesn't mean I can't get my point across and generate enthusiasm for my idea. I think it will be easier at our next meeting.

How likely (percent probability) do you feel your catastrophic expectation will occur the next time you are in this feared situation? *40 percent*

On a scale of 1 to 100, how intense was your distress about this feared situation before and after the exposure exercise?

Before: *85*   After: *40*

What do you need to learn now?

I still have some fear that my teammates will reject my ideas for a new game. They will be more critical when I mention that I want to make the hero in the game a flawed character. I know I will get some opposition to that, and I wonder if I will get so anxious that I won't be able to convince them that it's a great idea.

Note Helena's willingness to say something to her teammates that she knew some of them wouldn't like. This gave her a better chance to test her fearful expectation that she would perform poorly and be judged and rejected. Inspired by her debriefing, Helena immediately filled out her next Exposure Exercise Planning Form. As it turned out, her fearful arousal in her next team meeting dropped from 40 to 15 on her distress scale by the end of the exposure session. She was able to defend her flawed hero idea in spite of some strong objections. She estimated that the likelihood of her prediction of a catastrophic outcome in this feared situation dropped from 40 percent to 10 percent. She knew that she felt comfortable enough to continue giving presentations to her team without worrying about blowing it and being criticized and rejected.

Helena was ready to go back to question 5 on her Fear and Avoidance Assessment Form and pick another feared situation that she wanted to do, experience, or accomplish. From there she would once again go through the three steps of the exposure exercise: planning, exposure, and debriefing. At this point she had enough confidence to jump around to some of the highly feared situations on her list that she thought could teach her something useful, no matter how distressing she had rated them.

Research has shown that randomizing the challenge rather than moving from least to most fear-provoking situations actually makes for more rapid and long-lasting results (Craske et al. 2014). But if you find random exposures too stressful, move through your list of feared situations from the least to the most distressing, not going on to a more challenging fear situation until you have learned to face the fear situation below it. If you find that your exposures are not challenging enough, you can combine two of them that you have done before to make a challenging exposure. Right before your low-challenge exposure exercise, read an article about or watch a video of an example of what you fear.

Now it's time to plan and do your first exposure exercise, using the exposure exercise planning and debriefing forms. These forms are also available to download at http://www.newharbinger .com/43348.

Exposure Exercise Planning Form

Choose a feared situation you avoid or endure with distress:

_____

_____

Value (1–5): _____   **Distress level (0–100):** _____

Safety behaviors:

_____

_____

_____

_____

Catastrophic expectation of outcome:

_____

_____

_____

_____

Likelihood of your catastrophic expectation of outcome occurring: _____ percent

Your exposure exercise plan:

_____

_____

_____

_____

_____

Exposure Exercise Debriefing Form

Did what you were most worried about happen? No ( ) Yes ( )

How do you know? List specific evidence telling you that your feared outcome did or didn't occur.

_____

_____

_____

_____

What did you learn from doing this exposure exercise?

_____

_____

_____

_____

_____

How likely (percent probability) do you feel your catastrophic expectation will occur the next time you are in this feared situation? _____

On a scale of 1 to 100, how intense was your distress about this feared situation before and after the exposure exercise?

Before: _____   After: _____

What do you need to learn now?

_____

_____

_____

_____

_____

Special Considerations

Once you have successfully completed exposure exercises for all the examples on your feared situation list, it is recommended that you do an occasional booster session. A booster session consists of filling out an Exposure Exercise Planning Form, experiencing the exposure exercise, and filling out the Exposure Exercise Debriefing Form. This is particularly true if what you once feared and avoided is something that you rarely do for practical reasons, such as going on an airplane or swimming in the ocean. A booster session is also a good idea if you happen to have a frightening experience or you find yourself sliding back into your old avoidant habits.

Research shows that practice with facing your fear in a variety of different contexts makes for better outcomes (Craske et. al. 2014). Helena had the good fortune of being involved in several groups in which she could continue to practice public speaking after successfully completing this exposure program. She did still get nervous when she had to give a speech to large audiences at computer conventions, but she accepted this as natural. She felt confident that she could communicate her ideas well enough to be understood, and she no longer worried about being judged or rejected for her imperfect performance. She began traveling for work, which led her back to her Fear and Avoidance Assessment Form to tackle her fear of flying. She said that dealing with fear and avoidance, as with all stresses in life, was a journey, not a destination.

Further Reading

Craske, M. G., K. Kircanski, M. Zelikowsky, J. Mystkowski, N. Chowdhury, and A. Baker. 2008. "Optimizing Inhibitory Learning During Exposure Therapy." *Behaviour Research and Therapy* 46 (1): 5–27.

Craske, M. G., M. Treanor, C. Conway, T. Zbozinek, and B. Vervliet. 2014. "Maximizing Exposure Therapy: An Inhibitory Learning Approach." *Behaviour Research and Therapy* 58: 10–23.

Foa, E. B., and M. J. Kozak. 1986. "Emotional Processing of Fear: Exposure to Corrective Information." *Psychological Bulletin* 99 (1): 20–35.

McKay, M., M. Skeen, and P. Fanning. 2017. *The CBT Anxiety Solution Workbook: A Breakthrough Treatment for Overcoming Fear, Worry, and Panic.* Oakland, CA: New Harbinger Publications.

Wolpe, J. 1958. *Psychotherapy by Reciprocal Inhibition.* Palo Alto, CA: Stanford University Press.

CHAPTER 15

Anger Inoculation

In this chapter you will learn to:

- Relax rather than tense up in anger-provoking situations

- Develop coping thoughts to control anger-triggering cognitions

- Use provoking images to rehearse new coping skills and to inoculate yourself against anger

- Develop situation-specific anger coping plans

Background

Anger inoculation (McKay and Rogers 2000) is based on the anger management protocol developed by Jerry Deffenbacher (Deffenbacher and McKay 2000). The idea behind anger inoculation is that if you progressively expose yourself to memories of more and more provocative anger situations—while using coping skills—you will learn to manage the anger response. Raymond Novaco (1975) was the first to utilize this technique, and his research showed that it worked to reduce anger-driven aggression. Deffenbacher et al. (1987) confirmed Novaco's original findings, showing that combining relaxation and coping thoughts can significantly control anger. With anger inoculation, you learn to relax at the first sign of provocation and to counter your anger-triggering thoughts with thoughts intended to calm you and disconnect you from the upset. This training doesn't prevent you from feeling anger, but it gives you effective coping strategies, so you'll have the confidence that you can face a provocation without flying off the handle and damaging your relationships.

Anger inoculation involves four steps. They are as follows:

1. **Relaxation skills.** The specific relaxation training you'll need is available in other chapters of this book: diaphragmatic breathing, progressive relaxation, release-only relaxation, cue-controlled relaxation, and special place visualization.

2. **Coping thoughts.** You will create your own anger coping thoughts that will help you combat distorted thinking that triggers upsets.

3. **Inoculation.** You'll practice relaxation and cognitive coping skills while visualizing anger-evoking memories at five levels of intensity.

4. **Real-life coping.** You'll combine your most effective coping skills into an anger management plan designed for specific provocations.

Symptom-Relief Effectiveness

Novaco (1975), Hazaleus and Deffenbacher (1986), Deffenbacher et al. (1987), and Deffenbacher et al. (1990) have demonstrated across numerous studies that the anger inoculation protocol you'll learn here works to control the anger response. Significant reductions in both trait anger and anger incidents were achieved with this program.

Time to Master

You can master the key relaxation techniques in three to four weeks. Developing coping thoughts for specific anger situations would likely take several hours. The anger inoculation process in which you visualize provocative memories uses five levels of intensity with two anger images at each level. This work could take three to four weeks. Developing real-life coping plans may take an hour or two for each specific plan.

Instructions

Step 1: Learn to Relax

The fight-or-flight response is an important component of anger. Although angry thoughts may trigger the response, often you are already at a high level of sympathetic nervous system arousal when something happens that provokes angry thoughts and further stimulates your physiological arousal. This then, of course, produces more angry thoughts. An all too common example of this occurs when you are driving home in heavy traffic after a long day at work, suffering from a tension headache, and someone does something reckless. Already tense, you may lash out.

One way to intervene in your cycle of anger is to lower your overall sympathetic nervous system arousal through regular practice of deep relaxation techniques. But it also helps to use quick, breath-based relaxation strategies as soon as you start to feel upset. So, instead of shouting or blowing your car's horn and going crazy, you take several diaphragmatic breaths to release your pent-up tension.

The core relaxation skills you'll need to manage anger are all in this book. They are listed here—in the order you should learn them. It's hard to master cue-controlled relaxation without first learning progressive relaxation and release-only relaxation, so follow the sequence.

In provocative situations, some relaxation skills can be used quickly to get fast relief. Others are useful only as general stress relievers, and won't help you at the moment you're angry. Each technique is labeled as either "quick relief" or "general stress relief."

The skills you'll need are as follows:

- Diaphragmatic breathing (chapter 3)—*quick relief*

- Progressive relaxation (chapter 4)—*general stress relief*

- Relaxation without tensing, or release-only relaxation (chapter 7)—*general stress relief*

- Cue-controlled relaxation (chapter 7)—*quick relief*

- Special place visualization (chapter 6)—*general stress relief*

You will need to master or overlearn these relaxation techniques so that the quick relief strategies are available to you at a moment's notice. The general stress relief techniques provide you with deep release in two to three minutes. You must be able to relax with the same unconscious coordination with which you type or drive your car. Begin practice immediately. Do not go to step 3—anger inoculation—until you have mastered each of these relaxation skills.

Step 2: Develop Anger Coping Thoughts

Your thoughts have an enormous impact on your anger and your ability to defuse your anger. Anger-triggering thoughts are built on the following assumptions:

1. The belief that you have been harmed and/or victimized

2. The belief that the provoking person harmed you deliberately

3. The belief that the provoking person was wrong to harm you and should have behaved differently (McKay and Rogers 2000)

During stressful experiences, thoughts that paint you as a victim of deliberate and heedless harm will instantly ignite an anger reaction. And the more you think such thoughts, the angrier you will get.

Anger Distortions

Anger-triggering thoughts often distort reality. There are six key cognitive distortions that typically inflame anger, and one or more of them are likely to be factors in many of your anger experiences. Here are the six distortions:

1. **Blaming.** This is the belief that someone else is responsible for your pain, and there is nothing you can do about it. By blaming others, you forget that you have the power to make choices that will change the situation. You end up feeling helpless and stuck—waiting for someone else to fix things that will stay exactly as they are—until you do something. Another problem with blaming is that people are moving through life, trying to make the best choices they can to meet their own needs. When you blame others for their actions, you are blaming them for taking care of themselves in the best way they know how.

2. **Magnifying.** This is the tendency to take what is uncomfortable or unpleasant and frame it as so much worse. Words like "disgusting," "awful," "terrible," or "horrible" set you up to be angry because they exaggerate the impact of the provoking situation.

3. **Global labels.** These distortions use sweeping global judgments to inflame your anger. They paint the other person as totally bad, utterly worthless. Epithets such as "loser," "jerk," "bitch," "selfish pig," "bastard," and so forth are typical global labels. Their danger lies in ignoring the full reality of who the human being is with whom you are angry and reducing that person to a single negative term.

4. **Misattributions.** This distortion involves jumping to conclusions and mind reading. You assume malicious intent; you think you know people's motives and feelings toward you. You imagine that you can peer into others' hearts, seeing exactly why they do what they do. You don't ask questions or get direct feedback because that's too embarrassing, so you go on guessing and trying to read people, and a good part of the time you guess wrong.

5. **Overgeneralization.** This distortion uses words like "never," "always," "nobody," "everybody," and so on. "She's *always* late." "He's *never* willing to help." Overgeneralization makes an occasional occurrence feel like an ongoing event. The exaggeration makes everything feel intolerable and serves only to crank up your anger response.

6. **Demanding/commanding.** This distortion turns your personal needs or preferences into immutable laws—and when people ignore your preferences, you may feel as though they've broken one of the Ten Commandments. This gives you the right, it often seems, to really blast them. But there's one big problem with demanding/commanding. Often, other people don't agree with our definition of appropriate rules of conduct. They have their own rules, or at least their own interpretation of the rules, which leaves them feeling blameless while you think they've done wrong. Demanding/commanding is really nothing more than your values and needs imposed on others who may have very different values and needs.

Coping Thoughts

Each anger-provoking distortion requires a coping thought specifically designed to neutralize its effect. Here are some basic guidelines for developing these coping thoughts (adapted from McKay and Rogers 2000):

1. **Blaming**

   - Make a coping plan to solve the problem yourself.

   - Remind yourself that people are mostly doing the best they can to meet their own goals and needs.

   Example coping thoughts:

   Blaming only makes me feel helpless—what can I do to change the situation?

   My plan to change the situation is _____.

   I'm upset about this, but he/she is doing the best they can in the situation.

   They're doing what they need to do. I'll do what I need to do.

2. **Magnifying**

   - Be realistically negative (for example, the situation is disappointing or frustrating, not awful or horrible).

   - Answer this question: How bad is it really?

   - Restate using extremely accurate language.

   - Remind yourself of the whole picture—notice the positives as well as the negatives.

   Example coping thoughts:

   In the grand scheme of things, this is no big deal.

   This is a molehill-size problem. I don't have to make it bigger than it is.

   This is irritating, but it'll be history next week.

3. **Global Labels**

   - Be specific.

   - Describe the behavior, not the person as a whole.

   Example coping thoughts:

   Specifically what bothers me is _____.

Don't make it ugly, just state what the problem is.

Stick to the facts.

It's nothing more than a problem. I don't have to make him or her into a monster.

4. **Misattributions**

   - Remind yourself that you're guessing about motives—you don't know.

   - Find alternative explanations for the problem behavior.

   - Make a plan to check out your assumptions with the person who provokes you.

   Example coping thoughts:

   I'm guessing one possibility, but there are probably other reasons for _____'s behavior.

   Getting angry won't help me figure out what's going on. I need more facts.

   Some other possible reasons for this behavior are _____.

5. **Overgeneralization**

   - Revise your trigger thoughts so they don't include words like "always," "all," "every," and "never."

   - Use only specific and accurate descriptions.

   - Look for exceptions—recall how people sometimes behave very differently from their tendencies.

   Example coping thoughts:

   I'll just focus on the facts and I'll get through without blowing up.

   Be accurate—how often does this really happen?

   It doesn't always happen this way. There are lots of exceptions.

6. **Demanding/Commanding**

   - Focus on your desires and preferences—not *shoulds*. Think "I prefer," not "You should."

   - Figure out what needs the other person is meeting with his or her behavior.

   Example coping thoughts:

   I'm not getting what I want, but it's not the end of the world.

   I'd rather things were different, but I'll get through it.

People do what they want to do, not what I need them to do.

I wish this wasn't happening, but I can live with it.

Generalized Coping Thoughts List

If you find it difficult to develop your own coping thoughts, here's a list of coping thoughts for dealing with anger that may help. Many of these coping statements were developed in an anger management program that proved to be very effective (Novaco 1975).

- *Take a deep breath and relax.*

- *Getting upset won't help.*

- *Just as long as I keep my cool, I'm in control.*

- *Easy does it—there's nothing to be gained by getting mad.*

- *I'm not going to let them get to me.*

- *I can't change them with anger; I'll just upset myself.*

- *I can find a way to say what I want to say without anger.*

- *Stay calm—no sarcasm, no attacks.*

- *I can stay calm and relaxed.*

- *Relax and let go. There's no need to get my knickers in a twist.*

- *No one is right, no one is wrong. We just have different needs.*

- *Stay cool; make no judgments.*

- *No matter what is said, I know I'm a good person.*

- *I'll stay rational—anger won't solve anything.*

- *Let them look upset and foolish. I can act calm and in control.*

- *Their opinion isn't important. I won't be pushed into losing my cool.*

- *Bottom line, I'm in control. I'll get out of here rather than say or do something dumb.*

- *Take a time-out. Cool off, then come back and deal with it.*

- *Some situations don't have good solutions. Looks like this is one of them. No use getting all bent out of shape about it.*

- *Break it down. Anger often comes from lumping things together.*

- *Got angry, but kept the lid on saying dumb things. That's progress.*

- *Anger means it's time to relax and cope.*

- *If they want me to get angry, I'm going to disappoint them.*

- *I can't expect people to act the way I want them to.*

- *I don't have to take this so seriously.*

- *This is funny if you look at it that way.*

Step 3: Anger Inoculation

Now it's time to get to work. Think back and write down five anger situations you've struggled with over the past few weeks. List them in a journal or on a sheet of paper. Beneath each anger event you name, leave room to identify the following:

A. Your anger-triggering thoughts

B. Any anger distortions that might be embedded in your trigger thoughts

C. Counterresponse strategies (see previous section on coping thoughts) that might neutralize the distortion

D. One or more helpful coping thoughts—including revising the trigger thought to become more accurate

Example

Nancy, a forty-year-old schoolteacher, listed anger-provoking events in both her home and her classroom. Here are three of them:

Situation 1. Julian pulls out Rebecca's chair just when she's about to sit down—she falls on her back.

Anger-triggering thought: *He always does crap like this. He's a mean kid.*

Anger distortions: *Overgeneralization, global labeling.*

Counterresponse plan: *Stop using the word "always"; be specific; look for exceptions; focus on behavior, not the kid.*

Coping or revised trigger thought: *Julian gets in trouble maybe once a day. It's mostly silly stuff where he doesn't hurt anybody. And he's actually pretty sweet to the boy with cerebral palsy. I'm not gonna let his pranks get to me.*

Situation 2. I'm assigned yard duty for the second week in a row.

Anger-triggering thought: *They're always taking advantage of me because I don't complain. They're making this job unbearable.*

Anger distortions: *Overgeneralization, misattribution, blaming, magnifying.*

Counterresponse plan: *Stop using the word "always"; be specific; find alternative explanations; how bad is the job really?*

Coping or revised trigger thought: *This is only the second time in a year I've had to do two weeks in a row. It happens to other teachers, not just me. Maybe it's because Hilda was absent this week and they're shorthanded. It's just a hassle, nothing more, nothing less.*

Situation 3. Bill takes off for his poker night and leaves the dishes in the sink.

Anger-triggering thought: *He's so damned thoughtless. If you're going to go off and play, you'd better finish your work first.*

Anger distortions: *Global labeling, demanding/commanding.*

Counterresponse plan: *Focus on the behavior, not the person; stay with my desires and preferences, not "shoulds."*

Coping or revised trigger thought: *Bill sometimes forgets to do what he promised. I'd prefer he wouldn't leave a stack of dishes, but it's not the end of the world—he can do them when he gets home.*

On the next page is a worksheet for creating your own coping thoughts. Visit http://www.newharbinger.com/43348 to download this worksheet, so you can follow the steps for creating coping thoughts in any anger situation. Anger-triggering thoughts are those thoughts that set off your anger response.

Coping Thoughts Worksheet

1. Trigger thoughts that inflame my anger:

   a. _____

   b. _____

   c. _____

2. Anger distortions that underlie my trigger thoughts:

   a. _____

   b. _____

   c. _____

3. Counterresponse plan for each of my trigger thoughts (for example, looking for exceptions; alternative explanations; preferences, not shoulds; and so on). Revised trigger thought based on each counterresponse plan.

   a. Counterresponse plan: _____

   _____

   Revised trigger thought: _____

   _____

   b. Counterresponse plan: _____

   _____

   Revised trigger thought: _____

   _____

   c. Counterresponse plan: _____

   _____

   Revised trigger thought: _____

   _____

4. Helpful coping thoughts (see Generalized Coping Thoughts List earlier in this chapter):

   a. _____

   b. _____

   c. _____

Developed by McKay and Rogers (2000).

Visualizing Your Anger Scenes

Now it's time to practice your new coping skills (relaxation and anger coping thoughts) while visualizing anger scenes of increasing intensity. Let's start by selecting ten typical anger events that will help you rehearse what you've been learning.

To establish a hierarchy of gradually more provocative anger scenes, you can use a scale called Anger Units (AU), where 100 AUs is the worst rage you've ever felt in your life and 0 AUs is no anger at all. In the spaces provided below, write:

- Two mild-to-moderate anger scenes (40 to 50 AUs)

- Two moderate anger scenes (50 to 60 AUs)

- Two moderate-to-high anger scenes (60 to 75 AUs)

- Two high anger scenes (75 to 85 AUs)

- Two extreme anger scenes (85 to 100 AUs)

As you describe your anger scenes in Your Hierarchy of Anger Scenes worksheet, include details from the physical environment and what the provoking people are saying or doing. Also describe your trigger thoughts, feelings, and physical reactions.

Here's an example of one of Nancy's moderate-to-high anger scenes: "The school principal is presiding over a faculty meeting. It's hot, and I'm feeling flushed. She announces that I need to switch classrooms next year to something that's about the size of a broom closet. She's smiling in a phony, apologetic way. I'm thinking that she's taking my room away because I wouldn't do that demonstration reading project. What a bitch! I'm perspiring and my stomach's in a knot. I'm so angry, I want to let her have it, but I smother down the words."

Your Hierarchy of Anger Scenes

Mild to Moderate (40 to 50 AUs)

Scene 1: _____

_____

_____

Scene 2: _____

_____

_____

Moderate (50 to 60 AUs)

Scene 1: _____

_____

Scene 2: _____

_____

_____

Moderate to High (60 to 75 AUs)

Scene 1: _____

_____

_____

Scene 2: _____

_____

_____

High (75 to 85 AUs)

Scene 1: _____

_____

_____

Scene 2: _____

_____

_____

Extreme (85 to 100 AUs)

Scene 1: _____

_____

_____

Scene 2: _____

_____

_____

Anger Inoculation Protocol for Mild-to-Moderate and Moderate Anger Scenes

1. Create a Coping Thoughts Worksheet. Develop several anger coping thoughts prior to visualizing each scene.

2. Relax using cue-controlled relaxation and special place visualization. If there are specific areas of your body that remain tense, try progressive muscle relaxation or release-only relaxation.

3. Once you've relaxed, visualize the first anger scene at the mild to moderate level. Try to see as much detail as possible and hear whatever is being said. Intensify your anger response with some of your trigger thoughts. Keep at it, letting your anger rise as much as possible. Hold the scene in your mind for thirty seconds.

4. Now erase the scene and use your relaxation skills again. Also recall your anger coping thoughts. Keep this up until you feel calm again (0 AUs).

5. Repeat the whole sequence again, visualizing the second anger scene (at the mild-to-moderate level).

6. Alternate back and forth between these two scenes for four to six repetitions each. Then, using these same two scenes, have a second practice session a few days later.

7. Now move on to the two moderate anger scenes.

Anger Inoculation Protocol for Moderate-to-High Through Extreme Anger Scenes

For these higher-level anger scenes, you will make one important change in the procedure. Instead of erasing the scene after thirty seconds and beginning to cope (with relaxation and coping thoughts), *you'll use your coping skills while you continue to visualize the anger scene.* You will hold on to the provocative image while at the same time practicing cue-controlled relaxation and perhaps releasing tension in specific areas of your body. You will maintain the image while using your new coping thoughts or revised versions of trigger thoughts. Stay with the process until you feel completely calm (0 AUs).

After you've gotten down to 0 AUs in the first scene of a particular anger level, switch off the scene, do some cue-controlled breathing, and start visualizing the second scene. Switch back and forth between each scene four to six times, always waiting to get to 0 AUs before changing scenes. You are encouraged to do two practice sessions, switching scenes four to six times each, for each anger level.

It's hard to do two things at once (stay locked on an anger scene and, at the same time, cope). But with practice you can learn to do it. You'll soon be able to balance visualization with relaxation and anger management thoughts. Remember this: coping with real-life provocation is going to require this same balancing act. You'll need to deal with what's going on at the moment *and* use your coping skills. So all the practice you do now will put you in a far better position to handle real upsets.

Example

Let's go back to Nancy's anger scene with her principal—where she was being assigned to a "broom-closet" size classroom. Nancy begins by relaxing with her special place visualization (Tuolumne Meadows in Yosemite) and some cue-controlled relaxation. She notices any places in her body that feel tense, and she deliberately relaxes those areas. Now she begins to visualize the scene in the faculty meeting. She remembers her principal's phony smile as she told Nancy about her new classroom assignment. She recalls how hot the room felt and the flushed feeling in her body. She thinks, *What a bitch!*, and assumes that the principal is taking revenge for Nancy's refusal to do the demonstration project.

Now Nancy feels really steamed; this room assignment was a deliberate slap in the face. As her anger reaches the moderate to high level, Nancy begins to cope. She takes a cue-controlled breath; she reminds herself that her principal has done her favors as well as disappointed her. She thinks that the smaller room might reflect that her third-grade class is expected to have fewer students next year. While holding on to the scene of the faculty meeting and her principal's phony smile, Nancy reminds herself that *Getting upset won't change anything—stay cool.* She takes several more cue-controlled breaths.

Only when her anger is completely gone does Nancy switch off the scene. Now she returns for a few moments to her Yosemite Meadows before beginning her second moderate-to-high anger scene. Nancy continues to switch back and forth between her two moderate-to-high anger scenes four to six times.

Step 4: Real-Life Coping

Although you can't schedule real-life practice with provocations, you can prepare for them. You can have well-rehearsed coping thoughts ready, and you can stay alert for early warning signs of anger in your body and mind. The sooner you intervene with cue-controlled relaxation and coping thoughts, the more likely you are to maintain control.

If you know you are going to be in a situation that is likely to spark your anger, prepare your coping thoughts ahead of time and commit yourself to using them along with cue-controlled relaxation. With practice, this will be easier to do, and in time it will become more automatic. If you forget to use your coping skills, or you start to use them and then give up in the heat of the moment, visualize the scene later and practice coping just as you did when you were doing the anger inoculation exercises.

In addition to relaxation and using coping thoughts, it's always helpful to plan your best coping behaviors. What can you say or do to defuse the situation and get through it without blowing up?

Your Anger Plan

For each provocation where you forget to use your new skills, make a written anger plan. Visit http://www.newharbinger.com/43348 to download this Anger Coping Plan Worksheet.

Anger Coping Plan Worksheet

Precipitating event: _____

_____

_____

Anger-triggering thoughts: _____

_____

_____

Anger distortions: _____

_____

_____

Coping thoughts/revised distortions: _____

_____

_____

Relaxation strategy (Check for body tension? Cue-controlled breath? Diaphragmatic breath?):

_____

_____

_____

Coping behavior (Count to ten? Excuse yourself from the situation? Suggest a compromise? Validate both points of view?):

_____

_____

_____

Special Considerations

1. If you have difficulty following the relaxation protocol, you may want to record your relaxation routine and practice with that.

2. If you have difficulty forming images of anger scenes, include more sense impressions. For example, if your images are primarily visual, try to bring in sounds, smells, or the sense of touch. Add as many of these additional sensory elements to the scene as possible.

3. If you can imagine the anger scene clearly, but it produces little or no anger, focus more on anger-triggering thoughts. If that doesn't work, dump the scene and develop one that is more anger provoking. Or bring in a higher-level anger scene to work with.

4. If you are interested in learning more about irrational ideas that trigger unnecessary distress, refer to chapter 12, "Refuting Irrational Ideas."

Further Reading

Deffenbacher, J. L., and M. McKay. 2000. *Overcoming Situational and General Anger*. Oakland, CA: New Harbinger Publications.

Deffenbacher, J. L., K. McNamara, S. Stark, and P. M. Sabadell. 1990. "A Combination of Cognitive, Relaxation, and Behavioral Coping Skills in the Reduction of General Anger." *Journal of College Student Development* 31 (4): 351–58.

Deffenbacher, J. L., D. A. Story, R. S. Stark, J. A. Hogg, and A. D. Brandon. 1987. "Cognitive-Relaxation and Social Skills Interventions in the Treatment of General Anger." *Journal of Counseling Psychology* 34 (2): 171–76.

Hazaleus, S., and J. L. Deffenbacher. 1986. "Relaxation and Cognitive Treatments of Anger." *Journal of Consulting and Clinical Psychology* 54 (2): 222–26.

McKay, M., and P. D. Rogers. 2000. *The Anger Control Workbook*. Oakland, CA: New Harbinger Publications.

Novaco, R. 1975. *Anger Control: The Development and Evaluation of an Experimental Treatment*. Lexington, MA: D.C. Health.

CHAPTER 16

Goal Setting and Time Management

In this chapter you will learn to:

- Understand the limits of multitasking
- Clarify values, define your goals, and develop a plan to reach your goals
- Assess how you are currently spending your time
- Reorganize your time to fit your priorities
- Combat procrastination
- Use shortcuts for time management

Background

Most people approach the subject of time management with one major question: "How can I get more done in less time?" If you are one of these people, you are probably wondering how you are going to fit some of the exercises described in the other chapters of this book into your already overloaded schedule. You may feel so pressured to take care of the many demands and all the details in your life that you rarely have guilt-free time to do as you please. Or you may have loads of free time, yet you never get around to doing the things that would give you the most satisfaction. Other problems associated with ineffective time management include frequent lateness; low productivity, energy, and motivation; frustration; impatience; chronic vacillation between alternatives; difficulty setting and achieving goals; procrastination; lack of focus and purpose; and unproductive multitasking.

How is it that although each one of us has twenty-four hours in a day, some of us feel as though we have no time at all, while others manage to get their work done and still have enough time left over to enjoy themselves? People who manage their time effectively have learned to structure their lives so that they focus most of their time and energy on what is most important to them; they minimize the time they spend on activities they do not value. They realize that the quality of their lives is enhanced when they do a few things well instead of trying to find time to do a little of everything.

To realize the goals of effective time management, it is also important to look at how you can achieve balance in your life. Effective time management is a powerful way to lower your stress level, particularly when you use it to create balance in your life.

Limits of Multitasking

In today's world of information overload, people often think they can juggle phone calls, emails, text messages, and computer work to get more done. Unfortunately, multitasking is not as efficient as once thought, unless you're doing something mechanical such as your morning walk while listening to your favorite band through your earbuds. You simply delegate to your feet the task of walking while most of your attention is on music. But when you attempt to do two or more complicated tasks at once, multitasking can actually slow you down and cause you to make mistakes. Think about how stressful it is to write a report or learn new information while also having to respond to frequent interruptions. This is because your attention must rapidly shift back and forth between the two very different tasks. Each time you stop one task and begin another, you have to bring into focus the pertinent facts of the other task and get started with dealing with it. In the meantime, you may forget where you were in the first task, so it takes some time to reorient yourself before you can resume it. While some interruptions in your day are inevitable, this constant shifting back and forth not only wastes time and increases the possibility of errors but also adds to your stress.

So are you really being productive and safe when you:

- Talk on your cell phone while driving?

- Read email on your computer while you are talking to an important client on the phone?

- Plan a trip while using a skill saw?

- Respond to instant messages on your laptop while attending a meeting?

- Allow yourself to be interrupted while you are preparing an important report or focusing on an important decision?

The answer to these scenarios is an unequivocal no. Rather than trying to multitask, you will be more efficient and less stressed if you set aside inviolate time each day to focus on one thing and work without interruption.

In their 2004 book *The Power of Full Engagement*, the authors, Loehr and Schwartz, discuss the importance of balance in an age of overload. They state, "Being fully engaged means being able to immerse yourself in the mission you are on, whether it is grappling with a creative challenge at work, managing a group of people, spending time with loved ones, or simply having fun" (5).

The real key to time management is setting priorities and focusing on what you need to accomplish in the moment. This requires knowing what part of the day you have the most energy and planning your day around it. This includes doing routine tasks, for example, emailing or gardening, during low-energy periods and planning, writing, leading meetings, and learning new skills or content during higher energy periods.

The 80–20 Principle

If you are thinking "All of my responsibilities are important. I can't simply drop some of them to do what I please," consider the 80–20 principle. Vilfredo Pareto, an Italian economist, noted that 80 percent of what we gain comes from 20 percent of our effort; conversely, 80 percent of our effort produces only 20 percent of value. Empirical studies have shown this to be true time and again. This principle can be applied to many areas of life. For example, about 20 percent of the newspaper is worth your while to read. You are better off just skimming the rest of it. A good 80 percent of most people's mail is junk and best not read at all. The same applies to email; usually 20 percent requires your immediate response. Just about 80 percent of your housework can wait almost indefinitely, while 20 percent of it, if not done, would soon make your home uninhabitable.

In a 2008 article called "Managing Your Time When You Don't Have the Time," Barry J. Izsak, past president of the National Association of Professional Organizers, listed the following tactics for effective time management:

1. Focus on your priorities.

2. Be proactive, not reactive, with your time.

3. Plan your day.

4. Schedule your tasks.

5. Schedule appropriate tasks to the time and energy you have.

6. Don't procrastinate.

7. Don't be a perfectionist.

Symptom-Relief Effectiveness

Effective time-management skills can help with minimizing deadline anxiety, lack of focus, procrastination, and job fatigue.

Time to Master

You can begin to clarify what is most important in your life in as little time as an hour and then, as additional ideas come to you, return later to this important task. Defining your goals will take at least a few more hours. However, you can create an action plan for one of your goals in an hour. You will need at least three days to complete the time log.

Take at least several hours to evaluate how you actually spend your time—in terms of your priorities and goals—and decide how you want to change the way you spend your time, so that it more closely matches your ideals and goals. Although you can begin using the tips to combat procrastination and organize your time more efficiently within a week, you'll probably need several months of conscious effort before these techniques become habitual. If all this seems like a huge investment of your time, consider that the time you spend now will give you a lot more energy and free time in the future.

Instructions

In this chapter you will be asked to do six tasks:

1. Clarify your values.

2. Set goals.

3. Develop an action plan.

4. Evaluate how you spend your time.

5. Combat procrastination.

6. Organize your time.

Since each step builds on the previous ones, start with step 1 and work your way through to the last step.

Clarifying Your Values

The first step toward effective time management is deciding what is most worthwhile or desirable to you. People typically have priorities involving such things as career, health, home, family, spirituality, finances, leisure, learning, creativity, happiness, peace of mind, and communication. Knowing what is most valuable to you gives you direction in life. You can focus the majority of your time and energy on these values, rather than on other things that are less important to you. When you have to choose between alternatives, you can look to your priorities to help you make your decision.

Identify Your Highest Priorities

The following two brief guided fantasies can be done alone or with a family member or friend. They will help you identify your highest priorities.

1. Close your eyes, take a few deep breaths, and relax. Imagine yourself in a favorite place where you can take a few minutes to think. The time is many years from now. You have lived a long and full life. Reflect upon your life from this mature vantage point. What did you most enjoy experiencing and doing? What did you most appreciate accomplishing or having? Write your answers in this space or on a separate sheet of paper.

   _____

   _____

   _____

   _____

2. Return to your relaxed position and imagine yourself again in your favorite place. This time, you are still your current age. You have just learned that you have a rare illness that has no symptoms but will kill you in six months. Given only half a year to live, what do you want to experience, change, do, accomplish, and have? Write your answers in this space or on another sheet of paper.

   _____

   _____

   _____

   _____

Compare your two sets of answers. Are they the same or different? Most people actually faced with a life-threatening illness find that their priorities change. Things once believed to be crucial seem less important, and things once overlooked take on new meaning.

Order Your Values

Take the two lists that you developed in the previous exercise and order your values from the most to the least important.

1.	5.
2.	6.
3.	7.
4.	8.

You'll find that this list will come in handy when you have trouble choosing between two or more alternatives.

Here's how Alice, a single working parent, listed her values in order of importance.

1. *family*	5. *nice home*
2. *financial security*	6. *friends*
3. *health*	7. *travel*
4. *creativity*	8. *honesty*

Alice was troubled because her bosses were pressuring her to sign off on incomplete drafts of her designs. When she refused, they simply bypassed her signature. She vacillated between reporting her company's infractions to a government regulatory agency and remaining silent to avoid reprisal. When she examined her values, she realized that not speaking out was a form of dishonesty. But she also realized that although honesty was important to her, it had the lowest priority of all her values, and that all her other values were being successfully fulfilled by her job. With this insight, she stopped criticizing herself and waited until she had found a job in another company before reporting her former employer's misconduct. In that way she didn't jeopardize the other important aspects of her life.

Setting Goals

The second step to effective time management involves setting goals. Values are ideals. They are the things, experiences, qualities, and principles that you would most like to have in your life. Goals are real and specific. Goals are objectives that you want to achieve, given the constraints of your time and other resources. For example, your fondest hope might be to become a champion race-car driver. Your goal might be to cross the Indianapolis 500 finish line in first place three years from now. To bring your life into closer alignment with what you consider most worthwhile, use your list of values to guide you in defining your goals.

Designing Effective Goals

Here are five crucial questions to ask when designing effective goals:

1. **Is this a goal that you really want to devote a lot of time and energy to accomplish?** Or is it simply a dream of what you would like to have but are not willing to work for? Many people think that they would like to travel around the world, but they aren't willing to save the money this would require.

2. **Is this goal consistent with your highest values?** One reason you may not accomplish a goal is because it doesn't fit in with what is most important to you. If you value education and your goal is to finish college in the next year, but your highest priorities are family and socializing with friends, you may want to give yourself more time to complete college so that you won't have to neglect your family and friends.

3. **Is this goal achievable?** Is it specific enough so that you will know when you have achieved it? Is it achievable within a definite time frame that you can set for yourself? Do you have access to the resources necessary to achieve it? Instead of saying that you want to "retire on a comfortable income," set a date for retirement and specify an amount of money that you know you can realistically earn and save to support the lifestyle that you want when you retire. Note that you can modify your goals as you obtain more information.

4. **Is this goal positive?** You are far more likely to achieve goals you are moving toward rather than away from. For example, instead of setting the negative goal of no longer overeating, give yourself the positive objective of eating three sensible, nutritious meals a day.

5. **Are your goals in balance?** Do most of your goals involve your career and finances, while none or almost none of your goals have to do with health, relationships, or fun? Lack of balance is a major source of stress. If you spend your workday alone in front of a computer terminal, a useful, not too hard to achieve, short-term goal might be to get regular exercise outdoors with other people.

Balancing Your Goals

Do you have about an equal number of short-term, medium-term, and long-term goals? Some people plan on waiting until they retire to live their lives the way they really want to. Others can enjoy the here and now but are handicapped when it comes to achieving goals that involve delayed gratification. A mixture of short-term, medium-term, and long-term goals can provide you with satisfaction in the here and now as well as give you meaningful objectives to work toward.

Are your short-term and medium-term goals compatible with your long-term goals? If you want to live to a ripe old age to travel the world with old friends, your short-term and medium-term goals need to include taking care of your health, cultivating friendships, and making money.

Do you periodically reassess your goals to make sure that they are still what you want? As you work toward your goals, you gain new information and insights. Part of balancing your goals involves adapting them to the changes that invariably take place in life. Be flexible and allow yourself time to both reflect on and renew your goals.

Here's how Eric, a forty-one-year-old manager in an electronics firm, used his list of values to guide him in setting his life goals. First he listed his values:

1. Family: *To enjoy, take care of, and provide for them.*

2. Health: *To preserve the good health I enjoy into my eighties.*

3. Financial security: *To have enough money to take care of family, leisure, travel dreams, and retirement.*

4. Professional success: *To become a vice president with my company.*

5. Nature: *To spend time in the wilderness every year; to learn more about animal behavior.*

6. Friends: *To enjoy them by spending quality time with them and to help out.*

7. Spiritual: *To maintain my connection with my higher power and give my children an opportunity for this, too.*

8. Travel: *To go abroad as often and as far as my time and money permit.*

9. Communication: *To be open and honest with others and to know and feel that they are open and honest with me.*

10. Self: *To allow time to reflect on my life and to renew my focus on what is important to me.*

Here are the goals that Eric developed, based on his list of values.

Long-term goals (over five years):

1. *Own and live in a house on the lake where I spent my summers as a child.*

2. *Optimize my health with regular exercise, diet, rest, and medical checkups.*

3. *Raise my three children and provide each of them with an education.*

4. *Save and invest enough money so that I can retire at fifty-five years old, live at the lake, and travel.*

5. *Publish a book on hiking based on my wilderness experience.*

Medium-term goals:

1. *Become a vice president for the company in four years.*

2. *Buy a new house to accommodate our growing family within two years.*

3. *Find a church that the whole family can agree on and become an active participant.*

4. *Listen to audiobooks on personal financial planning and investing while commuting.*

5. *Go on a backpacking trip with friends to the Lost Coast a year and a half from now.*

Short-term goals:

1. *Go camping with my partner alone for a long weekend in the next month.*

2. *Set up a weekly family night starting this Thursday.*

3. *Have a fun evening with friends at least once a week.*

4. *Jog three mornings a week and take a hike with family and friends at least once a month.*

5. *Meditate for fifteen minutes before leaving the office to go home.*

6. *Remember to take a few deep breaths and relax my muscles when faced with a stressful event.*

7. *Take at least one week off from work once a quarter for renewal and to spend time hiking with my family and friends or alone.*

Writing Down Your Goals

Write down one or more specific goals for each of your priorities. You may find it helpful to list your various goals under the following three categories:

1. Your long-term goals (goals that will take you over five years to accomplish).

   _____

   _____

   _____

   _____

   _____

2. Your medium-term goals (goals that will take you between one and five years).

   _____

   _____

   _____

   _____

   _____

3. Your short-term goals (goals that will take from one week to less than one year).

   _____

   _____

   _____

   _____

   _____

Developing an Action Plan

Your third step is to identify the specific actions you need to take to achieve each of your goals. The most common reason that people do not attain their objectives is that they don't have an action plan that describes step by step how they are going to get from where they are now all the way to their goal. Without an action plan, your goal may seem too big and too remote. Without knowing what to do first, you may never get beyond the dreaming stage.

An effective action plan includes:

- A well-thought-out and specific goal

- A description of all the resources that you will need and how you will access them

- Each step you must take, in the correct order:

    - How you will monitor your progress

    - The most likely reasons you might procrastinate and how you will deal with this

    - What rewards you will use to motivate yourself

Here are two alternative strategies for creating an action plan.

Imagine That You've Already Achieved Your Goal

One strategy is to imagine that you've already achieved your goal. How would you feel, look, behave, and sound? How would the people around you respond to you? Once you have a clear picture of what you want and are in touch with the good feelings that picture generates for you, begin to work backward from that fantasized image. Ask yourself what steps you must have taken to achieve your objective. Notice which resources you used. Did you need to develop new skills? Did you use outside resources or did you simply rely on your personal ones? How much time did it take? How did you deal with obstacles like your fears and excuses and other people's demands on your time? How did you motivate yourself to keep going? Run a mental movie from where you are now all the way through to achieving your goal. Write down, in order, the steps you took.

Tom, a student in a college English class, used this approach. His goal was to receive an A on a paper for his creative writing class. First he visualized getting his paper back from his professor with an A on its cover. After relishing his pleasure and excitement and enjoying the imaginary congratulations of his friends, he went on to think through the steps he could have taken to reach that goal. Here's the list of steps that he generated:

1. *I take a walk by myself just to come up with a topic for my paper.*

2. *While walking, I come up with a great idea about writing a short story about salmon fishing in Alaska, which is how I earned money last summer. I reminisce about my experiences. I get excited about writing the paper.*

3. *I write an outline of my story.*

4. *I write a rough draft of my story.*

5. *I look over the rough draft and write a more polished version.*

6. *I ask my friend to read my paper. I'm encouraged by her positive comments.*

7. *I review and incorporate many of my friend's suggestions.*

8. *I make the final copy of my paper.*

9. *I turn my paper in on time.*

After thinking about his action plan, Tom realized that it didn't deal with one very familiar obstacle: his tendency to get sidetracked by his family and friends. He decided that his best strategy would be to reward himself with some time off to hang out with his friends once he had written a rough draft. Then he would bring himself back to his project by again visualizing accomplishing his goal.

Brainstorm

A second way to create an action plan would be to write your goal at the top of a blank sheet of paper and then randomly ask yourself questions about everything you need to know and do in order to achieve your objective. When you are finished brainstorming, rewrite the specific steps you need to take from where you are now all the way through to achieving your goal.

Angela's goal was to establish an ongoing aerobic exercise program for herself. She began by answering the following questions:

1. Why do I want to exercise?

   I want to feel and look healthy, fit, trim, and strong. One of my long-term goals is to be healthy into my old age.

2. How often and how long do I need to exercise aerobically to get the results I want?

   I need to do more research about exercise to answer these questions. I can talk to my friends about their experiences with exercise. I can read more. I want to start out gradually and set more challenging goals as I become stronger.

3. What kind of exercise do I like? What kind can I do and have the time and resources to do consistently?

   Walking, swimming, jogging, biking, and working out to an aerobic dance video are all good candidates.

4. What do I need in order to exercise safely and have a hassle-free time?

   I need a form of exercise that I can do without having to get in my car and deal with traffic. (That rules out swimming and biking!) There's a safe trail near my house. I have a DVD player, and I can buy an aerobic dance video. Except for shoes, I already have plenty of clothes I can dance, walk, and jog in.

5. *Which exercise video should I buy?*

   I can ask my friends for recommendations or rent online before choosing the one I like best.

6. What kind of shoes should I get and where do I find them?

   Go to the local sports store and ask the salesperson for help. I could read up on shoes, but I'd rather talk to my friends.

7. When am I going to exercise?

   After work, when I arrive home, before I do anything else.

8. How am I going to motivate myself to stick with this program?

   I can jog with a friend. I can participate in local races. I can pay attention to how much better I feel and look when I have been exercising regularly for a while. I can reward myself with new exercise clothes and videos and gold stars. I can always do aerobic dance, even when the weather is bad or it's dark outside, because it's so enjoyable.

9. How am I going to monitor my progress?

   I will keep track of my progress by reviewing the gold stars on my calendar every other week with my friend Stacey, who knows what I am trying to accomplish and is very supportive of me.

Here's the action plan that Angela developed after she read through and reorganized her answers:

1. *Define my specific exercise goal and keep in mind my purpose in exercising regularly.*

2. *Read more about aerobic exercise to find out how often and how long I need to exercise.*

3. *Talk to my friends about jogging, proper shoes, and aerobic dance videos.*

4. *Find a jogging partner. (This is an optional step: not essential for me to start my program.)*

5. *Consult with a salesperson at a local sports store and buy a comfortable pair of shoes to fit my exercise needs.*

6. *Try out aerobic videos by renting or borrowing them first.*

7. *Buy favorite aerobic videos online or at a local bookstore.*

8. *Jog or work out to aerobic dance videos when I get home right after work.*

9. *Monitor my progress by putting a gold star on the days of the week that I exercise. I'll use the calendar in my kitchen, since I look at it every day.*

10. *Evaluate my progress with Stacey.*

11. *Reward myself by buying new exercise clothes, participating in local races, and buying new videos. I can look and feel great!*

Evaluating Your Progress

Identifying a way to keep track of your progress should be a part of your action plan. One powerful approach is to plan to go over what you have accomplished toward your goal with a support person every couple of weeks. Choose someone who understands and appreciates what you are trying to do. This person should be able to give you positive suggestions and encouragement as well as point out when you may be fooling yourself.

By your second two-week progress evaluation, you should begin to see some positive results. Success can serve as a powerful reinforcer to continue your program, but don't let your first gains trick you into slacking off. Old habits don't die easily, and it can take three or more months to develop new ones.

If you are not seeing positive results or you catch yourself making excuses for not following through on your plan, don't be too hard on yourself. Instead, reassess your original goal. Is this what you really want? If not, modify your goal. If it is something you want, consider how you can modify your action plan to start moving toward your goal.

Evaluating How You Spend Your Time

Now you can begin the fourth step toward effective time management by keeping a daily log of your time. Do this in real time, rather than at night trying to estimate how much time you spent on the various activities that filled your day. Most people tend to grossly underestimate how long it takes them to do their various tasks, and they also tend to overlook or forget the unplanned activities that pop up during the day.

If you really want to learn something new about yourself, stop once an hour during the day to record how long it took you to do each activity that you were involved in during that hour. At the very least, get out your notebook after lunch and dinner and before bed and write down every activity you engaged in. Note the amount of time each one took. When you're through, the total amount of time for all activities should be fairly close to the total number of hours you were awake. You can also use the Your Time Log included here. Visit http://www.newharbinger.com/43348 to download this worksheet.

Keep recording all of your activities for this time inventory for at least three days. Categories of activities at work might include paperwork, email or instant messaging, phone calls, socializing face-to-face, meetings, multitasking, low-priority work, focused productive work, interruptions, eating, and/or conference calls. Typical activities unrelated to work are personal hygiene, grooming, dressing, cooking, eating, naps, daydreaming, child care and parenting, shopping, household chores and maintenance, commuting, travel for errands, personal telephone calls, face-to-face conversations, watching television, engaging in hobbies or reading, participating in sports, exercising, and other recreation. Modify or add categories to suit yourself.

Keep in mind that this time log is designed to help you break down and examine as carefully as you need to the various ways that you use your time so that you can decide later whether you want to spend more or less time engaged in each of these activities.

Before keeping a daily log, you may want to look at Samantha's Time Log. Samantha, a radio public-affairs interviewer, kept this record on the first day of her three-day time assessment.

Your Time Log

Activity	Time
Waking through lunch	
After lunch through dinner	
After dinner until sleep	

Samantha's Time Log

Activity	Time
Waking through lunch	
Lying in bed trying to get up	20 minutes
Shower	20 minutes
Grooming and dressing	25 minutes
Cooking breakfast	5 minutes
Eating breakfast and reading paper	10 minutes
Phone call (family)	10 minutes
Commute and listen to news	45 minutes
Morning staff meeting (10 minutes late)	40 minutes
Routine work—review and respond to:	60 minutes
Phone messages	
Electronic mail	
Written memos	
Mail	
Daydreaming	5 minutes
Socializing (friend)	15 minutes
Meeting (15 minutes late)	45 minutes
Productive work (preparing for interview)	40 minutes
Lunch with friend (15 minutes late)	75 minutes
After lunch through dinner	
Productive work (preparing for interview)	95 minutes
Phone call (friend)	5 minutes
Daydreaming	10 minutes
Low-priority work (helping coworker)	65 minutes
Socializing with coworker	15 minutes
Phone call (work related)	30 minutes
Commute and listen to news	45 minutes
Shopping	40 minutes
Mail	10 minutes
Phone call (personal)	25 minutes
Neighbor visits	20 minutes
Phone call (work related)	30 minutes
Cook while listening to news on TV	60 minutes
Eat	20 minutes

After dinner until sleep	
Clean up kitchen	15 minutes
Phone call (personal)	10 minutes
Television (documentary)	60 minutes
Reading novel	25 minutes
Turn off light (30 minutes late)	

Evaluating Your Time Log

Now that you know how you are actually spending your time, you are ready to compare the inventory you made with your real priorities. From there, you'll be able to decide what changes you want to make to bring your current schedule into closer alignment with your most important values and goals. Here are some questions that will guide you in making this comparison.

1. **Which of the activities on your daily log are in line with your values and goals?**

    Mark these activities with a star.

    Samantha starred "reading paper" and "listen to news," since these activities reflected her priority of staying current with the news. She starred her productive time at work preparing for radio interviews because this reflected her priority to be a successful radio interviewer. She starred "phone call (friend)" since one of her priorities was to spend time with friends.

2. **Which of the activities on your daily log are not in line with your values and goals?**

    Circle these activities.

    Samantha was amazed to find that on this day she had spent so much time preparing, eating, and cleaning up after meals. She felt that she had spent too much time on the phone and reading and responding to email and text messages for work. She also realized that she had wasted a half hour in the morning with extra time in bed and a long shower. She recognized that she allowed unexpected calls and socializing to get in the way of being on time. When she analyzed her work patterns, it became obvious that her most productive hours were at midday—and that lunch was a big interruption right in the middle of this time.

Look at the circled items on your list and write down how you would be willing to reschedule, reduce, or eliminate low-priority activities in your day.

_____

_____

_____

_____

_____

3. **Are any of your values being violated by any of the activities on your daily log?**

Mark these activities with an X.

Engaging in activities that run counter to your values can cause you to feel guilty, ashamed, anxious, depressed, resentful, or exhausted. Samantha's problem with tardiness ran counter to her priorities of peace of mind and being a successful radio interviewer. She felt rushed, anxious, guilty, and embarrassed when she arrived at meetings late.

Look at the items that you've marked with an X and write down how you would be willing to change your behavior so that it no longer violates your values.

_____

_____

_____

_____

_____

4. **Are some of your values and goals being neglected or ignored?**

Activities that reflect these neglected values and goals may be the very ones that you need to expand or increase to bring balance into your life. On the other hand, these neglected values actually may have a lower priority at this time in your life than your other values, and you may realize that you feel okay about postponing activities associated with them.

Samantha noticed that her priorities having to do with friends, family, and health were underrepresented in how she spent her time. Except for brief phone calls, she didn't talk with her family. Since her parents and sisters lived in another state and she had recently visited them, this limited contact was okay with her for right now. She did want to spend more time with friends and take better care of herself physically. Her sedentary lifestyle and eating habits had caused her to gain weight.

Write down how you would be willing to change your behavior so that it would be consistent with the values and goals that you have been neglecting.

_____

_____

_____

_____

_____

Samantha decided that she was willing to make the following immediate changes in her use of time:

1. *Eat a quick breakfast that does not require cooking.*

2. *Prioritize being on time over answering unexpected phone calls and other low-priority activities.*

3. *Limit reading and responding to email to twice a day.*

4. *Limit lunch to an hour and take it later in the day to take advantage of my most productive time of day.*

5. *Prepare simple dinners in half an hour.*

6. *Limit most work-related calls to ten minutes.*

7. *Skim written communication for "must know" and "must respond" information.*

8. *Prioritize going to sleep on time over watching TV and reading.*

9. *Get up with the alarm and limit shower to ten minutes.*

10. *Go to the gym and work out with friends four nights a week.*

Although it is unlikely that you would want to try to do something that reflects each one of your values and goals every single day, you can integrate all of your values and most of your goals into your activities if you plan your time on a weekly or even monthly basis. Continue using the tools you learned earlier in this chapter to clearly define your goals and prepare an action plan that lets you evaluate and reward yourself for the progress you've made.

Combating Procrastination

The fifth step toward managing your time more effectively is to get yourself unstuck. What distasteful activity are you avoiding? Compare it with your values. Does it violate one of your priorities? If it does, are you ready to take a stand and declare that you are not going to do it? If not, what can you do to change your circumstances in the future so that you will no longer violate one of your values? If you are avoiding an activity that is tied to one of your goals, review the section in this chapter on setting effective goals. If you don't know where to start, create an action plan. If you simply need to get better organized, refer to the sixth and final step in this chapter, which deals with organizing your time.

Here are ten additional suggestions to use when you find yourself procrastinating.

1. **Stop worrying.** You probably spend more time worrying about chores that you do not want to do than you would spend by simply doing them. To illustrate this point to yourself, keep track of how much time it takes you to complete each distasteful task.

2. **Start small.** Once you start doing an unpleasant task, you may find that it isn't as bad as you anticipated. Lead yourself into the cold water with a small but related task. For example, if you have to mow the lawn, decide to go as far as filling the gas tank on the mower and wheeling it out to the edge of the lawn.

3. **Count the cost.** Make a list of all the unpleasant aspects of doing the activity you are avoiding and then make a second list of the consequences of putting it off. Look squarely at the discomfort of doing it versus the cost of delay and ask yourself which list contains the greater degree of unpleasantness. Use this information to create enthusiasm for getting the job done.

4. **Look for the hidden rewards.** Look for any payoffs you may be receiving for not getting the distasteful job done. For example, by procrastinating you may be avoiding feeling anxious or facing the possibility of failure. Also examine the advantages of avoiding whatever changes might follow from completing the task. For example, success might mean that you lose the attention that you now get from people who nag you or sympathize with your predicament.

5. **Confront negative beliefs.** Read chapter 12, "Refuting Irrational Ideas," to confront beliefs that may be interfering with doing what you need to do. Are you making statements to yourself like "No way am I going to do this, it just isn't fair," "I must do it perfectly," "Life should be easy," "I can't stand the thought of giving a speech in front of a group of strangers," "What if I succeed? They'll expect even more out of me," or "I'll fail, so why even try?"

6. **Double your resistance.** Exaggerate and intensify whatever you are doing that puts off beginning a task. If you stare at yourself in the mirror in the morning instead of getting to work, draw that stare out. Really examine all of your pores and go over each quadrant of

your face minutely. Keep it up until you are really bored and getting to work seems like a more attractive alternative.

7. **Take responsibility for each delay.** You are the one wasting your precious time. Make a list of each procrastination or escape activity and note how long each took. Add up the total and list all the positive things you could have done with that time if you'd simply begun and finished the job.

8. **Tie a distasteful activity to an activity that you know you will do.** For example, if you dislike exercise, find a gym you can visit on your way home from work, or plan to exercise by walking to lunch at a restaurant twenty minutes from your office.

9. **Reward yourself for doing activities that are unpleasant to you.**

10. **Finish things.** Avoid beginning a new task until you have completed a specific segment of your current task. The experience of finishing something is itself a great reward.

Organizing Your Time

The sixth and final step toward more effective time management is to become better organized. Here are eleven suggestions to structure your time and focus your attention on creating the life of your choice.

1. **Use an organizer app on your phone, tablet, or computer, or purchase a notebook organizer.** Find one that includes a daily, weekly, and monthly calendar and use it.

2. **Make sure that your list of daily goals and your calendar reflect your long-term, medium-term, and short-term goals.** You can schedule time each day for exercise and for practicing relaxation techniques. If spending quality time with a loved one is a high priority, block off regular time on your calendar to do this and include that time on your daily to-do list. If you arrange your schedule of activities on a weekly or even monthly basis, you will find that you have time to work on all of your important goals.

3. **Plan for efficiency.** Combine activities that can be done at the same time, such as watching your favorite TV show while exercising, ironing, or washing dishes. Use a digital video recorder to record favorite TV shows, so you can watch them at a convenient time. You can sequence activities to save time. Match tasks to your varying energy levels. Although you can usually predict your energy level at different points during the day and plan accordingly, occasionally you will run out of steam earlier than anticipated. If so, you may want to reschedule activities that require energy and alertness to a time when you can perform them with maximum efficiency.

4. **Minimize time wasters.** Cut back on TV, time spent on the Internet, telephone interruptions, drop-in visitors, unproductive meetings, ineffective delegation of responsibilities, crises, activities that lack direction, and overly ambitious goals. Plan ways to avoid as many predictable time wasters as possible, but be realistic enough to schedule some time for unexpected interruptions.

5. **Learn to say no.** Set limits on how much you are willing to do for others. If you have difficulty with this, see chapter 17, "Assertiveness Training."

6. **Make a list of things to do when you're waiting.** Good candidates include doing a relaxation exercise, planning tomorrow's list of goals, reviewing your priorities and goals, reading a book, or filing your nails.

7. **Set aside several short periods each day for quiet time.** Use this time to practice your deep relaxation techniques. This will help you stay in touch with what is most important to you rather than rushing faster and faster in response to others' demands.

8. **When you are performing a high-priority activity, focus your full attention on it.** Make a list of your usual distractions and plan how you can block each one of them. For instance, if you often find yourself daydreaming when you should be working, schedule in a visualization session or some other way of using your imagination during one of your quiet times.

9. **Arrange your environment to support your values and goals.** If your priorities require focus and concentration, make sure that you have a quiet room or corner available for reading, writing, practicing deep relaxation, or just thinking through your plans.

10. **Don't waste time on decisions that involve equally attractive or inconsequential alternatives.** If you find yourself in a quandary over choices like this, just flip a coin and go with the winning call.

11. **Reward yourself for improving your time management.** One of the greatest rewards of effective time management comes from not having to rush to accomplish the important things in your life. By prioritizing and planning your activities, you can choose to move through your day at a more leisurely pace.

Organizing Your Day

Managing your time on a daily basis requires setting immediate priorities and sticking to them. At the beginning of each day, develop a to-do list that reflects your goals as well as the necessary tasks. Then sort the activities you've listed into the following categories:

1. *Top drawer.* These are the most essential and most desired items.

2. *Middle drawer.* You could put these activities off for a while, but they are still important.

3. *Bottom drawer.* You can easily put these tasks off indefinitely with no harm done.

Go through your list and mark each item TD, MD, or BD according to its status.

Now, when you start your day, you have a blueprint for how to apportion your time. Start with the top-drawer items first and then work your way down the list. Move on to the middle drawer only when all of your top-drawer items have been completed. If you have too many top-drawer tasks to finish in a day, then you've given too many things a high priority. Assign top-drawer status only to tasks that absolutely cannot be put off and would result in negative consequences if they were.

Banish the bottom-drawer items from consideration unless you have completed all your higher priority items for the day. The definition of bottom-drawer items is that they can wait. Unless it's your boss who's asking, keep away from commitments that force you to spend time in the bottom drawer. Be prepared to say "I don't have the time" to these requests. If circumstances force you to take on a bottom-drawer task, try to delegate it. Give it to your assistant, your housecleaner, or your children.

As you move through your day, stay focused on high-priority tasks and make sure to limit your opportunities for procrastination. Block off any escape routes that turn up: you can schedule daydreaming for a later time and put off socializing until a chunk of work is done. Avoid getting caught up in busywork or less important errands, and resist the impulse to run out for coffee or any other tempting indulgences.

At the end of the day, review your to-do list. Check off the items that you completed as planned and give yourself a mental pat on the back. Add anything you did that was not on your original list. Note whether it was a high-, medium-, or low-priority item. Important things you did not finish can be moved to the next day. A good time to prepare a day's list of goals is the preceding evening or first thing in the morning. Either way, you start out fresh, on top of things, and in tune with your priorities.

Track and Manage Interruptions

How often do you allow yourself to be interrupted by others? How often do you take on a new task not on your top-drawer list? Interruptions may be phone calls, people who drop by your office or home, or getting involved in someone else's agenda or priority for the day.

To see how often you let yourself be distracted by daily interruptions, keep a notebook handy, and when this happens, begin to track how you react and what you could do differently in the future.

Here are several tips on how to manage interruptions in your day:

- Schedule time during your day to take care of email, voice mail, phone calls, and receiving visitors.

- Be proactive in reaching out to personal or business relationships and check in to assess and anticipate needs before those needs become priorities; for example, get regular status reports from important clients, employees, or an aging parent. These check-ins can be done by telephone, email, or text instead of face-to-face meetings.

- When you are interrupted, make it clear that you have only a few minutes and that you will be able to get back to the person at a later, specific time.

You will discover that balance, focus, and renewed energy are but three of the benefits of clarifying your values, priorities, and goals. Managing your time efficiently is a path that will help you regain a sense of control and purpose in your life. Enjoy your new journey!

Further Reading

Covey, S. R. 2004. *The 7 Habits of Highly Effective People.* Revised ed. New York: Simon & Schuster.

Griessman, B. E. 1994. *Time Tactics of Very Successful People.* New York: McGraw-Hill.

Izsak, B. 2008. "Managing Your Time When You Don't Have the Time." https://www.selfgrowth.com/articles.

Loehr, J., and T. Schwartz. 2004. *The Power of Full Engagement: Managing Energy, Not Time, Is the Key to High Performance and Personal Renewal.* New York: Simon & Schuster.

Manhart, K. 2004. "The Limits of Multitasking." *Scientific American Mind* 14 (15): 62–67.

McCorry, K. J. 2005. *Organize Your Work Day in No Time.* New York: Que Publishing.

Morgenstern, J. 2004. *Never Check E-Mail in the Morning: And Other Unexpected Strategies for Making Your Work Life Work.* New York: Fireside.

Rubinstein, J. S., D. E. Meyer, and J. E. Evans. 2001. "Executive Control of Cognitive Processes in Task Switching." *Journal of Experimental Psychology: Human Perception and Performance* 27 (4): 763–97.

Stautberg, S. S., and M. L. Worthing. 1992. *Balancing Acts! Juggling Love, Work, Family, and Recreation.* New York: Master Media.

CHAPTER 17

Assertiveness Training

In this chapter you will learn to:

- ■ Evaluate your current patterns of communication

- ■ Differentiate between aggressive, passive, and assertive styles of communication

- ■ Examine mistaken traditional assumptions and your assertive rights

- ■ Express your feelings and opinions, set limits, and initiate change

- ■ Use nonverbal assertive communication

- ■ Listen assertively

- ■ Avoid manipulation

Background

Andrew Salter (1949) initially described assertiveness as a personality trait. It was thought that some people had it and some people didn't, just like extroversion or stinginess. But Wolpe (1958) and Lazarus (1966) redefined assertiveness as expressing personal rights and feelings. They found that nearly everybody could be assertive in some situations and yet be totally ineffectual in others. The goal of assertiveness training is to increase the number and variety of situations in which assertive behavior is possible and to decrease occasions of passive collapse or hostile blowup.

You are assertive when you stand up for your rights in such a way that the rights of others are not violated. Beyond just demanding your rights, assertiveness implies that you can: express your personal likes and interests spontaneously; talk about yourself without being self-conscious; accept compliments comfortably; disagree with someone openly; ask for clarification; and say no. In short, when you are an assertive person, you can be more relaxed in interpersonal situations.

Some people think that assertiveness training turns nice people into irascible complainers or calculating manipulators. Not so. It's your right to protect yourself when something seems unfair. You are the one who best understands your discomfort levels and your essential needs.

How you interact with people can be a source of major stress. Assertiveness training can reduce that stress by teaching you to stand up for your legitimate rights without bullying others or allowing them to bully you. You can use assertive communication to reduce conflict and build strong, supportive relationships.

Before reading any further, write down how you would typically respond to the following problem situations:

1. You finish shopping in the market, and after you walk out you discover that the change is three dollars short.

   I would: _let it be and walk out_

2. You order a rare steak and it arrives medium-well done.

   I would: _Just eat the steak_

3. You're giving a friend a lift to a meeting. The friend keeps puttering around for half an hour and you realize that you will arrive late for the meeting.

   I would: _Tell the friend to hurry up_

4. You've been looking forward all week to seeing a particular movie, and your companion informs you that he wants to see a different movie.

   I would: _Convince him to go watch the other movie_

5. You're relaxing watching TV after a long, hard day. Your spouse pops in, list in hand, and says, "I thought you'd never get here. Quick, go out and pick up these things from the store."

I would: ___Absolutely not_____

_____

_____

6. While you wait for the clerk to finish with the customer ahead of you, another customer comes in and the clerk starts to wait on her before you.

I would: ___Just wait until the clerk comes to me_____

_____

_____

After you have written down what you would do in these problem situations, set your responses aside. They will be put to use shortly.

Investigators such as Jakubowski-Spector (1973) and Alberti and Emmons (2008) have demonstrated that people who show relatively little assertive behavior do not believe that they have a right to their feelings, beliefs, or opinions. In the deepest sense, this means rejecting the idea that we are created equal and are meant to treat each other as equals. Believing this, they can't find grounds for objecting to exploitation or mistreatment. Most likely such people learned as children some traditional assumptions that implied their perceptions, opinions, feelings, and wants were less important or less correct than those of others. They grew up doubting themselves and looking to others for validation and guidance.

When you were a child, you didn't have much choice about which traditional assumptions you were taught. Now, however, you have the option of deciding whether to continue behaving according to assumptions that keep you from being an assertive adult. Each of the following mistaken assumptions violates one of your legitimate rights as an adult:

Mistaken Traditional Assumptions	Your Legitimate Rights
1. It is selfish to put your needs before others' needs.	You have a right to put yourself first sometimes.
2. It is shameful to make mistakes. You should have an appropriate response for every occasion.	You have a right to make mistakes.
3. If you can't convince others that your feelings are reasonable, then the feelings must be wrong, or maybe you are going crazy.	You have a right to be the final judge of your feelings and accept them as legitimate.
4. You should respect the views of others, especially if they are in a position of authority. Keep your differences of opinion to yourself. Listen and learn.	You have a right to have your own opinions and convictions.
5. You should always try to be logical and consistent.	You have a right to change your mind or decide on a different course of action.
6. You should be flexible and adjust. Others have good reasons for their actions and it's not polite to question them.	You have a right to protest unfair treatment or criticism.
7. You should never interrupt people. Asking questions reveals your stupidity to others.	You have a right to interrupt in order to ask for clarification.
8. Things could get even worse, don't rock the boat.	You have a right to negotiate for change.
9. You shouldn't take up others' valuable time with your problems.	You have a right to ask for help or emotional support.
10. People don't want to hear that you feel bad, so keep it to yourself.	You have a right to feel and express pain.
11. When someone takes the time to give you advice, you should take it very seriously. They are often right.	You have a right to ignore the advice of others.
12. Knowing that you did something well is its own reward. People don't like show-offs. Successful people are secretly disliked and envied. Be modest when complimented.	You have a right to receive formal recognition for your work and achievements.

13. You should always try to accommodate others. If you don't, they won't be there when you need them.	You have a right to say no.
14. Don't be antisocial. People will think you don't like them if you say you'd rather be alone than spend time with them.	You have a right to be alone, even if others would prefer your company.
15. You should always have a good reason for what you feel and do.	You have a right not to have to justify yourself to others.
16. When someone is in trouble, you should help them.	You have a right not to take responsibility for someone else's problem.
17. You should be sensitive to the needs and wishes of others, even when they are unable to tell you what they want.	You have a right not to have to anticipate others' needs and wishes.
18. It's always a good policy to stay on people's good side.	You have a right not to always worry about the goodwill of others.
19. It's not nice to put people off. If questioned, give an answer.	You have a right to choose not to respond to a situation.

As you continue working through this chapter, keep in mind that assertive communication is based on the assumption that you are the best judge of your thoughts, feelings, wants, and behavior. Nobody is better informed than you are regarding how your heredity, history, and current circumstances have shaped you into a unique human being. Therefore, you are the best advocate for expressing your positions on important issues. Because of your uniqueness, there are many times when you differ with significant people in your life. Rather than overpowering the meek or giving in to the aggressive, you have the right to express your position and try to negotiate your differences.

Symptom-Relief Effectiveness

Assertiveness training has been found to be effective in dealing with depression, anger, resentment, and interpersonal anxiety, especially when these symptoms have been brought about by unfair circumstances. As you become more assertive, you begin to lay claim to your right to relax and take better care of yourself.

Time to Master

Some people master assertiveness skills sufficiently for symptom relief with just a few weeks of practice. For others, several months of step-by-step work are needed to experience significant change.

Instructions

Step 1: Identifying Three Basic Interpersonal Styles

Assertiveness is a skill that can be learned, not a personality trait that some are born with and others are not. The first step in assertiveness training is to identify the three basic styles of interpersonal behavior.

- **Aggressive style.** In this style, opinions, feelings, and wants are honestly stated but at the expense of someone else's feelings. The underlying message is "I'm superior and right, and you're inferior and wrong." The advantage of aggressive behavior is that people often give aggressive individuals what they want in order to get rid of them. The disadvantage is that aggressive individuals make enemies, and people who can't avoid them entirely may end up behaving dishonestly toward them in order to avoid confrontations.

- **Passive style.** In this style, opinions, feelings, and wants are withheld altogether or expressed indirectly and only in part. The underlying message is "I'm weak and inferior, and you're powerful and right." The advantage of passive communication is that it minimizes responsibility for making decisions and the risk of taking a personal stand on an issue. The disadvantages are a sense of impotence, lowered self-esteem, and having to live with the decisions of others.

- **Assertive style.** In this style, you clearly state your opinions, feelings, and wants without violating the rights of others. The underlying assumption is "You and I may have our differences, but we are equally entitled to express ourselves to one another." The major advantages include active participation in making important decisions, getting what you want without alienating others, the emotional and intellectual satisfaction of respectfully exchanging feelings and ideas, and high self-esteem.

To test your ability to distinguish interpersonal styles, label person A's behavior in the following scenes as aggressive, passive, or assertive:

Scene 1

A: Is that a new dent I see in the car?

B: Look, I just got home, it was a wretched day, and I don't want to talk about it now.

A: This is important to me, and we're going to talk about it now.

B: Have a heart.

A: Let's decide now who is going to pay to have it fixed, when, and where.

B: I'll take care of it. Now leave me alone, for heaven's sake!

A's behavior is   ☐ Aggressive   ☐ Passive   ☐ Assertive

Scene 2

A: You left me by myself at that party… I really felt abandoned.

B: You were being a party pooper.

A: I didn't know anybody—the least you could have done was introduce me to some of your friends.

B: Listen, you're a grown-up. You can take care of yourself. I'm tired of you nagging to be taken care of all the time.

A: And I'm tired of your inconsiderateness.

B: Okay, I'll stick to you like glue next time.

A's behavior is   ☐ Aggressive   ☐ Passive   ☐ Assertive

Scene 3

A: Would you mind helping me for a minute with this file?

B: I'm busy with this report. Catch me later.

A: Well, I really hate to bother you, but it's important.

B: Look, I have a four o'clock deadline.

A: Okay, I understand. I know it's hard to be interrupted.

A's behavior is   ☐ Aggressive   ☐ Passive   ☐ Assertive

Scene 4

A: I got a letter from Mom this morning. She wants to come and spend two weeks with us. I'd really like to see her.

B: Oh no, not your mother! And right on the heels of your sister. When do we get a little time to ourselves?

A: Well, I do want her to come, but I know you need to spend some time without my relatives underfoot. I'd like to invite her to come in a month, and instead of two weeks, I think one week would be enough. What do you say to that?

B: That's a big relief to me.

A's behavior is   ☐ Aggressive   ☐ Passive   ☐ Assertive

Scene 5

A: Boy, you're looking great today!

B: Whom do you think you're kidding? My hair is a fright, and my clothes aren't fit for the Goodwill box.

A: Have it your way.

B: And I feel just as bad as I look today.

A: Right. I've got to run now.

A's behavior is   ☐ Aggressive   ☐ Passive   ☐ Assertive

Scene 6

While at a party, A tells her friends how much she appreciates her boyfriend taking her out to good restaurants and to the theater. Her friends criticize her for being such an old-fashioned, unliberated woman.

A: Not so. I don't make nearly as much at my job as he does at his. I couldn't afford to take us both out or pay my own way to all the nice places we go. Some traditions make sense, given the economic realities of both of our lives.

A's behavior is   ☐ Aggressive   ☐ Passive   ☐ Assertive

Now that you have labeled person A's responses in these scenes as aggressive, passive, or assertive, compare your assessment with ours:

Scene 1. A is aggressive. A's seemingly innocent question is actually an accusation in disguise. A's insistence on immediate action with total disregard for B's state of mind sets up a polarized conflict in which B is likely to withdraw and feel wrong and defensive.

Scene 2. A is aggressive. The tone is accusing and blaming. B is immediately placed on the defensive and no one wins.

Scene 3. A is passive. A's timid opening line is followed by complete collapse. The file problem must now be dealt with alone.

Scene 4. A is assertive. The request is specific, nonhostile, and open to negotiation.

Scene 5. A is passive. A allows the compliment to be rebuffed and surrenders to B's rush of negativity.

Scene 6. A is assertive. She stands up to the prevailing opinion of the group and achieves a clear, nonthreatening statement of her position.

Step 2: The Assertiveness Questionnaire

The second step in assertiveness training is to identify those situations in which you want to be more effective. Having clarified the three interpersonal styles, now reexamine your responses to the six problem situations presented at the beginning of this chapter. Label your responses as falling primarily in the aggressive, passive, or assertive style. This is a start in objectively analyzing your behavior and finding out where assertiveness training can most help you.

To further refine your assessment of the situations in which you need to be more assertive, complete the following questionnaire, adapted from Sharon and Gordon Bower's 2004 book *Asserting Yourself*. Put a check mark in column A by the items that are applicable to you and then rate those items from 1 to 5 in column B:

1. Comfortable
2. Mildly uncomfortable
3. Moderately uncomfortable
4. Very uncomfortable
5. Unbearably threatening

(Note that the varying degrees of discomfort can be expressed whether your inappropriate reactions are hostile or passive.)

	A Check here if the item applies to me	B Rate from 1–5 for discomfort
WHEN do I behave nonassertively?		
Asking for help	√	1
Stating a difference of opinion	√	3
Receiving and expressing negative feelings		
Receiving and expressing positive feelings	√	3
Dealing with someone who refuses to cooperate	√	4
Speaking up about something that annoys me	√	4
Talking when all eyes are on me	√	2
Protesting a rip-off		
Saying no	√	2
Responding to undeserved criticism	√	4
Making requests of authority figures	√	2
Negotiating for something I want	√	1
Having to take charge	√	2
Asking for cooperation	√	1
Proposing an idea		
Asking questions		
Dealing with attempts to make me feel guilty	√	2
Asking for service		

Asking for a date or an appointment		
Other		
WHO are the people with whom I am nonassertive?		
Parents		
Fellow workers, classmates	√	2
Strangers	√	∧
Old friends	√	2
Spouse or mate		
Employer		
Relatives		
Children		
Acquaintances	√	2
Salespeople, clerks, hired help	√	∧
More than two or three people in a group	√	3
Other		
WHAT do I want that I have been unable to achieve with nonassertive styles?		
Approval for things I have done well		
To get help with certain tasks		
More attention, or time with my mate		
To be listened to and understood		
To make boring or frustrating situations more satisfying		

	A Check here if the item applies to me	B Rate from 1–5 for discomfort
To not have to be nice all the time	✓	3
Confidence in speaking up when something is important to me	✓	3
Greater comfort with strangers, store clerks, mechanics, and so on		
Confidence in asking for contact with people I find attractive		
To get a new job, ask for interviews, raises, and so on	✓	2
Comfort with people who supervise me or work under me		
To not feel angry and bitter a lot of the time		
To overcome a feeling of helplessness and the sense that nothing ever really changes		
To initiate satisfying sexual experiences		
To do something totally different and novel		
To have time by myself		
To do things that are fun or relaxing for me		
Other		
WHY am I hesitant to be assertive?		
If I'm assertive, I am concerned that I might appear to be:		
Selfish	✓	4
Imperfect or foolish	✓	4
Wrong or crazy	✓	3
Disrespectful	✓	4

Illogical or inconsistent	✓	3
Inflexible		
Stupid	✓	4
A troublemaker		
A complainer	✓	4
Unappreciative	✓	4
A show-off	✓	3
Uncooperative	✓	3
Uncaring	✓	3
Insensitive	✓	4
Unfriendly	✓	4
Rude	✓	4
Weak*	✓	2
Other		

*Aggressive people worry about being taken advantage of, not getting what they want, and not being obeyed if they are perceived as weak.

Adapted from Bower, S., and G. Bower. 2004. *Asserting Yourself: A Practical Guide for Positive Change.* New York: Da Capo Press.

Evaluating your responses. Now, examine your answers and analyze them for an overall picture of what types of situations and people threaten you. How does nonassertive behavior contribute to the specific items you checked on the *What* list? In constructing your assertiveness program, it will be useful to initially focus on items you rated as falling into the 2 to 3 range. These are the situations that you will find easiest to change. Items that are very uncomfortable or threatening can be tackled later.

If you checked off any of the items on the *Why* list that address your concerns about appearing in a negative light if you are assertive, review the Mistaken Traditional Assumptions and Your Legitimate Rights, from which the items on the *Why* list were derived. Remember that you are your own best advocate and that you have a responsibility to take care of yourself even when you don't have the full approval or support of others.

It's natural to feel anxious when you are doing something new. With practice, you will feel more comfortable behaving assertively. You may not always get what you want when you are assertive, inasmuch as other people also have the right to disagree and say no, but you are much more likely to achieve your goals when you behave assertively rather than passively or aggressively. Chapter 12, "Refuting Irrational Ideas," is another resource that can help you examine unhelpful self-talk that contributes to your discomfort with being assertive.

Step 3: Describing Your Problem Scenes

The third step in assertiveness training, according to Sharon and Gordon Bower (2004), is to describe your problem scenes. Select a mildly to moderately uncomfortable situation that suggests itself from items on the Assertiveness Questionnaire. Write out a description of the scene, being certain to include *who* the person involved is, *when* it takes place (time and setting), *what* bothers you, *how* you deal with it, your *fear* of what will take place if you are assertive, and your *goal*. Always be specific! Generalizations will make it difficult later on to write a script that will make assertive behavior possible in this situation. The following is an example of a poor scene description.

> *I have a lot of trouble persuading some of my friends to listen to me for a change. They never stop talking, and I never get a word in edgewise. It would be nice for me if I could participate more in the conversation. I feel that I just let them run over me.*

Notice that the description doesn't specify *who* the particular friends are, *when* this problem is most likely to occur, *how* the nonassertive person acts, what *fears* are involved in being assertive, and a specific *goal* for increased involvement in the conversation. This scene might be rewritten as follows:

> *My friend Joan (who), when we meet for a drink after work (when), often goes on and on—nonstop—about her marriage problems (what). I just sit there and try to be interested (how). If I interrupt her, I'm afraid she'll think I just don't care (fear). I'd like to be able to change the subject and talk sometimes about my own life (goal).*

Here is a second poor scene description:

> *A lot of times I want to strike up a conversation with people, but I worry that maybe they don't want to be disturbed. Often I notice someone who seems interesting, but I can't imagine how to get their attention.*

Once again there is a lack of detail. No clear statement is made as to *who* these people are, *when* the experience takes place, *how* the nonassertive person behaves, or the specific *goal*. The described scene will become much more useful by including the following elements:

There is an attractive girl (who) who always brings a bag lunch and often sits at my table in the cafeteria (what, where) at lunch (when). I just eat in silence and read my book (how). I would like to start a conversation by asking about her boss, who has a very hard-to-get-along-with reputation (goal), but she looks so intent on her book, I'm afraid she will think that I am rude and be annoyed if I interrupt her (fear).

As you write three or four problem scenes, you will likely recall the thoughts and feelings you actually experienced. You might notice, for example, that in each problem scene you shoot yourself down with negative thoughts (*I can't do it… I'm blowing it again…boy, do I look stupid*), or you usually feel tense in the stomach and seem to be breathing way up in your chest. Other chapters of this workbook offer some strategies that may help you cope with distressing habitual thoughts and physical reactions when you act assertively. Refer to "Refuting Irrational Ideas," "Relieving Worry and Anxiety," "Facing Fear and Avoidance," "Anger Inoculation," "Applied Relaxation Training," and "Breathing" (diaphragmatic breathing). This chapter, however, primarily focuses on changing your habitual way of behaving in these problematic interpersonal situations.

Step 4: Your Script for Change

The fourth step in assertiveness training is writing your script for change. A script is a working plan for dealing with the problem scene assertively. There are five elements in a script:

1. **Arrange a time and place to discuss your problem that is convenient for you and for the other person.** For example, "After we have dinner tonight in the living room, I will ask my roommate if she would be willing to talk about keeping the living room tidy. If she doesn't want to do it then, I'll ask her to name a more convenient time." This step may be excluded when dealing with spontaneous situations in which you choose to be assertive, such as when a person cuts ahead of you in a line of waiting people.

2. **Define the problem situation as specifically as possible.** This is essential for focusing the discussion. Here is your opportunity to state the facts as you see them and share your opinion and beliefs without attacking the other person. For example: "I notice that your clothes, books, and papers are left out in the living room for days at a time. We live in a small apartment, and when one person doesn't clean up after herself, the place gets messy fast."

3. **Describe your feelings so that the other person has a better understanding of how important the issue is to you.** Once your feelings are expressed, they can often play a

major role in helping you get what you want, especially when your opinion differs markedly from that of your listener. If nothing else, the listener may be able to relate to and understand your feelings about an issue even when she or he totally disagrees with your perspective. When you share your feelings, you become less of an adversary. There are three useful rules to remember when assertively expressing your feelings:

a. Do not substitute an opinion for a feeling ("I feel that you're a lazy, immature slob!"). More accurate feeling statements are "I hate living in a messy house. I resent having to clean up after you in order to have a neat living room."

b. Use *I-messages* that express your feelings without evaluating or blaming others. Rather than saying "You are inconsiderate" or "You piss me off," you would say "I'm annoyed and frustrated."

c. Use I-messages to connect the feeling statement with specific behaviors of the other person. For example, "I feel angry and frustrated when you leave your things in the living room for days at a time." Contrast the clarity of this message with this vague blame statement: "I feel pissed off because you are so inconsiderate."

4. **Express what you want in one or two easy-to-understand sentences.** Be specific and firm. Instead of expecting others to read your mind and magically meet your needs, as in the case of the passive individual, clearly state your wishes and needs. Rather than assuming that you are always right and entitled to getting your way, as an aggressive person might, state your wants as preferences, not as commands. For example, "I would like you to not leave clothes, books, and papers in the living room when you are not using them."

5. **Reinforce the other person to give you what you want.** The best reinforcement is to describe positive consequences. "We will have a neater living room… We'll save money… We'll have more time together… I'll give you a backrub… My mother will stay only one week… I'll be less tired and more fun to be with… I'll be able to get my work in on time… Little Julia will do better in school," and so on.

In some cases, describing positive consequences may be ineffective. If the person you're dealing with seems resistant or if you feel that you're having trouble motivating him or her to cooperate with you, consider describing some negative consequences for failure to cooperate. The most effective negative consequences are descriptions of the alternative way you will take care of yourself if your wishes aren't accommodated.

- "If we can't leave on time, I'll have to leave without you. Then you'll have to drive over later by yourself."

- "If you can't clean the bathroom, I'll hire someone to do it once a week and add it to your rent."

- "If you won't fold and put away your clothes, I'll just leave them in this box. I guess you can sort through it whenever you need something."

- "If you keep talking in this loud, attacking way, I'll leave. We can talk again tomorrow."

- "If you get drunk at the party, I'm driving home."

- "If your check bounces again, we'll have to work on a cash-only basis."

- "If you keep talking during the movie, I'm going to ask the manager to come over here and deal with the problem."

- "If you can't give me an accurate idea of when you'll be home, I'm not going to cook dinner and keep it warm for you."

Notice that these examples are different from threats. The consequence of noncooperation is that the speaker takes care of his or her interests. The consequences are not designed to hurt but are merely to protect the speaker. Threats usually don't work, because they make people so angry. If you do make a threat ("You won't go to my sister's wedding? I won't go to your family reunion!"), be sure you are willing and able to back it up. Even then, the threat will often do more harm than good.

As an example of a script for change, let's say that Jean wants to assert her right to have half an hour every day of uninterrupted peace and quiet while she does her relaxation exercises. Frank often interrupts with questions and attention-getting maneuvers. Jean's script goes like this:

Arrange a time and place to discuss the situation:

I'll ask Frank if he's willing to discuss this problem when he gets home tonight. If he isn't, we'll set a time and place to talk about it in the next day or two.

Define the problem specifically:

At least once, and sometimes more often, I'm interrupted during my relaxation exercises—even though I've shut the door and asked for the time to myself. My concentration is broken and I find that relaxing deeply is harder.

Describe your feelings using I-messages:

I feel angry when my time alone is broken into, and I feel frustrated that the exercises are then made more difficult.

Express what you want simply and firmly:

I would like not to be interrupted when my door is closed unless it's a dire emergency. As long as the door is closed, assume that I am still doing the exercises and want to be alone.

Reinforce the other person to give you what you want:

If I'm not interrupted, I'll come in afterward and chat with you. If I am interrupted, I will take more time to do the exercises.

In the next example, Nick demonstrates how to use the assertive script for change to say no. Nick has felt very reluctant to approach his coworker to tell her he has changed his mind about helping with her new project. Nick's script is as follows:

Arrange a time and a place to discuss the situation:

I'll send an email tomorrow morning requesting a time to talk about this problem.

Problem:

Clara, I know that I agreed to help you with your new project, but I have discovered that it's taking much more time than I anticipated. I'm finding that I'm not getting my own work done, and that's going to cause me big problems with my boss.

Feelings:

I feel guilty about changing my mind and letting you down. I'm also feeling pressured and anxious about falling behind in my own work when a deadline is looming.

Wants:

I'm going to have to take myself off your project sometime in the next week. Is Friday too soon?

Reinforcement:

I might be available to help you in a smaller capacity after the end of the fiscal year next month. In the meantime, consider asking Jeff to help you out, since he is between projects now.

(Note: Nick doesn't have to offer a reinforcement to make his withdrawal from the project more acceptable to Clara, but he chooses to because he is willing to help her as long as his own work doesn't suffer, and he wants to maintain a good working relationship with her.)

Now, here is an example of how you can use a script for change when a situation suddenly presents itself and you want to be assertive. You skip arranging a time. Before you speak, think of a sentence or two to complete the three essential elements of the script for change. Offer a reinforcement if you like.

Crystal is watching TV in the family room when her little brother comes into the room, grabs the remote, and starts channel surfing. Crystal stifles her first response to call him "an inconsiderate little creep" and to wrestle the remote away from him. After thinking about the four basic elements of her script for change, she says, "*Lenny, I was watching my favorite program when you came in here and started channel surfing* [problem]. *I'm really annoyed that you turned off the program I was watching without consulting with me first* [feeling]. *I want you to turn back to my program right now* [want]. *If you do that, I'll leave the TV to you for the rest of the evening when my program is over in fifteen minutes* [positive reinforcement]."

Exercise: Read the following script for change. Then, in the space provided, write down what you think is wrong with it, and rewrite the script based on what you've learned about good scripts for change.

For the past two semesters, Julie has wanted to take a night class in ceramics. Each time her husband had an excuse about why he could not watch the children on the night of the class. Here's Julie's script for change:

Arrange a time and a place to discuss the situation:

When Kevin gets home tonight.

Problem:

You've made it impossible for me to take my ceramics class for a whole year. I've been pushed around for too long.

Feelings:

I'm sick and tired of you being such a selfish, inconsiderate son of a gun.

Request:

You're just going to have to suffer through babysitting while I take my class.

Reinforcement:

If you don't like it, you can kiss this marriage good-bye.

Problems with this script for change:

1. _____

   _____

   _____

2. _____

   _____

   _____

3. _____

   _____

   _____

4. _____

   _____

   _____

5. _____

_____

_____

Compare your ideas with the following problems we found in Julie's script for change:

1. She didn't get an agreement on the time and place for the discussion.

2. She used nonspecific and blaming phrases such as "made it impossible" and "pushed around."

3. She failed to specify exactly what her husband was doing that was a problem.

4. She accused her husband of being a selfish, inconsiderate son of a gun rather than expressing her feelings about his specific undesirable behaviors.

5. She did not specify which nights during the semester she needed her husband to do the child care or how long the semester would last. Instead, she made a very unappealing demand.

6. She threatened negative consequences that she probably would not be willing to carry out.

Now, rewrite Julie's script for change so that she is being assertive:

Arrange a time and a place for discussion:

_____

_____

Problem:

_____

_____

Feelings:

_____

_____

Request:

_____

_____

Reinforcement:

_____

_____

Here is an example of how Julie might make her request:

Arrange a time and a place:

I'll ask Kevin if he would be willing to talk after breakfast Saturday morning about doing the child care during my ceramics night class. If he's not, I'll ask him to name a time in the immediate future when he is.

Problem:

I've missed two previous ceramics classes because you weren't available for child care on class night. I've waited a year and I would like to enroll this time.

Feelings:

I feel frustrated that I haven't been able to explore something that really excites me. I also feel hurt and angry when you do other things rather than help me take the class.

Request:

I'd like you to look after the children on Wednesday nights between 6:30 and 9:00. The class starts January 25th and ends June 2nd.

Reinforcement:

If you're willing to do this for me, I'll cook your favorite meatloaf for you on Wednesdays, but if you're not, we'll have the expense of a babysitter.

In the new and improved script for change, the time to talk is agreed upon, the described problem behavior has become specific, the expressed feelings are now nonthreatening I-messages tied to specific behaviors, and the request is simple and concrete. Julie's reinforcements are realistic and explicit. Note that negative reinforcement is often not necessary, and that positive reinforcement may require no more than the assurance that you will feel good if a certain behavior change is made. Elaborate promises usually can be avoided.

Exercise: Now, you can write your own scripts for change. Download the Script for Change form at http://www.newharbinger.com/43348 so that you can write out different scripts for change.

Script for Change

Arrange a time and a place to discuss the situation (if appropriate):

_____

_____

_____

Define the problem specifically:

_____

_____

_____

Describe your feelings using "I-messages":

_____

_____

_____

Express your request simply and firmly:

_____

_____

_____

Reinforce the other person to give you what you want (if you like):

_____

_____

_____

Step 5: Assertive Nonverbal Communication

The fifth step in assertiveness training is to learn to use your body and tone of voice to support your assertive words. Practicing your assertive scripts for change in front of a mirror or with a friend will help you master the following five basic rules:

1. Maintain direct eye contact. Note that it is natural to blink and look away occasionally.

2. Maintain an erect body posture.

3. Speak clearly, calmly, and firmly.

4. Don't whine or use an apologetic or hostile tone of voice.

5. Use gestures and facial expressions for emphasis that are congruent with what you have to say, such as a serious look rather than a smile when you are saying no to a door-to-door salesperson.

Exercise: Rehearse your written scripts in front of a mirror, using assertive nonverbal communication. Be your own coach: observe what you are doing well and what you might improve next time.

Exercise: Record your rehearsals to further refine your assertive voice.

Exercise: Practice your script with a friend who can play the role of the other person. Afterward, ask your friend's opinion on what you did well and what you might do to improve when you express your script for change in real life.

Exercise: Use your script for change in a real-life situation. Afterward, ask yourself what you did well, and how you could do better if you were to do it again. Did you get the response you wanted from the other person? If you didn't, give yourself credit for trying to stand up for yourself. Continue to rehearse and then use your scripts for change in real life, adding in new assertiveness skills as you learn them.

Step 6: Assertive Listening

The sixth step of assertiveness training involves learning how to listen. As you practice being assertive in real-life situations, you will find that sometimes you need to deal with an issue that is important to the other person before he or she will be able to focus on what you have to say. This is especially true when what you want directly conflicts with long unspoken and unmet needs of the listener.

For example, it might be wise to practice assertive listening if your spouse responds to your request for change with *"You want an hour of silence when you get home from work? Well, I haven't said this before, because you're working so hard, but I'm ready to tear out my hair after spending the entire day with the kids. I have needs too, you know."*

In listening assertively, you focus your attention on the other person so that you can accurately hear the speaker's opinions, feelings, and wishes. Assertive listening involves three steps:

1. **Prepare.** Become aware of your feelings and needs. Are you ready to listen? Are you sure that the other person is really ready to speak?

2. **Listen and clarify.** Give your full attention to the other person; listen to the speaker's perspective, feelings, and wants. If you are uncertain about one of these three elements, ask the speaker to clarify with more information: *"I'm not quite sure how you view the situation… could you say more about it? How do you feel about this? I don't understand what you want… could you be more specific?"*

3. **Acknowledge.** Communicate to the other person that you heard his or her position. For example, you might say, *"I hear you don't want to take on this new project, because you're feeling overwhelmed with your current responsibilities and want to catch up."* Another way to acknowledge the other person's feelings is to share your feelings about what has already been said: *"I'm feeling overwhelmed too, and I feel terrible about having to ask you to do more work."*

Assertive listening and assertive expressing go together. Here is a sequence in which both people use assertive listening and expressing skills to solve a problem. John is unhappy about the way Carmen communicates her needs to him.

John: Is this a good time to talk about something that's bugging me a little? (*Arrange*)

Carmen: Okay.

John: Yesterday you told me you were feeling cut off and kind of abandoned by me. (*Problem*) I felt like I was doing something horrible to you. I felt very wrong, but totally confused about what exactly I was doing. (*Feelings*) Rather than making such generalized complaints like that, could you say what I'm not doing that you need, or what I could change? (*Request*) I think I could be a lot more responsive that way. (*Reinforce*)

Carmen: What was it you needed more information about? (*Clarify*)

John: What you needed me to do, at that moment, to feel closer.

Carmen: Okay, so what you're saying is that when I talk about my feelings without making any specific requests for change, it leaves you feeling confused and responsible. (*Acknowledge*)

John: Right.

Carmen: Well, sometimes I'm just telling you how I feel. I don't know why I feel that way or what to do about it. Telling you is an attempt to open the discussion. (*Redefining problem*)

John: I see. So you really aren't sure what I could do at that point. (*Acknowledge*) How about just saying you aren't sure and asking what we could do about it together? Making it "we" instead of just me would help a lot on my end. (*New request*)

Carmen: That sounds right. I like it.

Notice that Carmen clarifies and acknowledges before attempting any further explanation of the problem from her point of view. Then, in a nonblaming way, she explains why she can't go along with John's request. John, in turn, acknowledges what Carmen has said. He then uses this new information to make a second proposal that works better for Carmen.

But here's the rub: You can't always expect the other person to play by the rules. There are times when you'll have to both express and listen assertively in the face of defensive or hostile reactions. Consider Hal and Sara's case:

Sara: I have a problem with the cash projections. Can we talk? (*Arrange*)

Hal: Whatever.

Sara: Currently you're only running them out for the next three months, and I can't see how sales, inventory, and costs are going to interact six to eight months down the line. (*Define*) I'm getting pretty nervous about the big printing bills because we don't know if the money will be there. (*Describe feeling*) Could you run out the cash projection for at least six months? (*Express request*) I think we'd all breathe easier. (*Reinforce*)

Hal: Forget it, Sara. There's no time. I haven't got the bodies in my department to do stuff like that. Take a Valium and cool out.

Sara: How much extra work would it take? (*Clarify*)

Hal: Forget it, Sara. (Loudly) Forget it, okay?

Sara: I hear you. You're overworked and haven't the staff to take on anything extra. (*Acknowledge*) But I'm wondering, how many extra hours of work are involved? (*Clarify*)

Hal: At least twenty. Keep pushing, Sara. I'm up to here with everybody's demands.

Sara: I hear how stressed you are. (*Acknowledge*) If once a month I got a twenty-hour bookkeeper from the pool for you, could you handle it? (*New request*)

Hal: Probably. Let me see the body first, Sara.

In the face of sarcasm and anger, Sara continues to clarify and acknowledge until she understands Hal's problem. Hostile resistance doesn't sidetrack her. She keeps working to understand Hal's stresses and needs so she can make a new, more acceptable proposal.

Exercise: Role-play assertive listening with a friend. Have your friend play the role of a real person in your life who isn't ready to hear your script, because he has issues of his own that are getting in the way. Use assertive listening to help him express his problems, feelings, and wants. Alternatively, write out a dialogue as you imagine it taking place between you (the assertive listener) and the other person (the expresser).

Exercise: Practice assertive listening in everyday life with or without combining it with a script for change. Be sure the other person wants to express the issue.

Step 7: Arriving at a Workable Compromise

The seventh step of assertiveness training is learning how to arrive at a workable compromise. When two people's interests are in direct conflict, a fair compromise that totally satisfies both parties is difficult, if not impossible, to achieve. Instead, look for a workable compromise you both can live with, at least for a while. Although a compromise might emerge naturally in your discussion, sometimes you and the other person might have to make a list of all the alternative solutions you can think of. Cross off the list those that aren't mutually acceptable. Finally, decide on a compromise you can both live with. This brainstorming process is most effective if you let your imaginations run wild while you are generating ideas. It's best to agree to review a workable compromise in a specified length of time, such as a month. At that time, you can examine the results of your changed behavior. If you aren't both sufficiently satisfied, you can renegotiate and fine-tune your compromise.

Typical compromise solutions include the following:

- *My way this time, your way next time.*

- *I get part of what I want and you get part of what you want.*

- *Meeting halfway.*

- *If you'll do _____ for me, I'll do _____ for you.*

- *We'll do this one my way, but we'll do _____ your way.*

- *We'll try my way this time, and if you don't like it, you can veto it next time.*

- *We'll try your way this time, and if I don't like it, I can veto it next time.*

- *My way when I'm doing it, your way when you're doing it.*

If you feel resistant to brainstorming and making lists of alternatives, try this simpler approach. When someone doesn't want to give you what you want, ask for a counterproposal. If the counterproposal isn't acceptable to you, make a new one of your own. But first do a little assertive listening to uncover the other person's feelings and needs in the situation. Keep going back and forth with counterproposals until something works for both of you.

A second route to compromise asks this question: *"What would you need from me to feel okay doing this my way?"* The answer may surprise you and offer solutions you never thought of.

Exercise: Plan how you will use a workable compromise in a situation where you are in conflict with another person. Combine it with your script for change and assertive listening.

Step 8: Avoiding Manipulation

The eighth and final step to becoming an assertive person is learning how to avoid manipulation. Inevitably, you will encounter blocking gambits from those who seek to ignore your assertive requests. The following techniques are proven ways to overcome the standard blocking gambits.

Broken record. When you find that you are dealing with someone who won't take no for an answer or refuses to grant you a reasonable request, you can carefully choose a concise sentence to use as your broken-record statement that you'll say over and over again. For example, you could say to your insistent four-year-old, "Jeff, I am not going to give you any more candy." You might say to the aggressive used-car salesman, "I am not going to buy a car today; I'm just looking." You could say to the uncooperative store clerk, "I want you to give me back my money for this defective radio." Briefly acknowledge that you have heard the other person's point, and then calmly repeat your broken-record statement without getting sidetracked by irrelevant issues. "Yes, but... Yes, I know, and my point is... I agree, and... Yes, and as I was saying... Right, but I'm still not interested."

Content-to-process shift. Shift the focus of the discussion from the topic to an analysis of what is going on between the two of you. "We're getting off the point now." "We've been derailed into talking about old issues." "I realize I'm doing all the talking. I get the impression you don't feel comfortable talking to me about this right now. Am I right?"

Defusing. Ignore the content of someone's anger and put off further discussion until they have calmed down. "I can see that you are very upset and angry right now. Let's discuss it later this afternoon."

Assertive delay. Put off a response to a challenging statement until you are calm, have more information, or know exactly how you want to respond. "Yes very interesting point... I'll have to reserve judgment on that... I need more time to think about the issue... I don't want to talk about it at this time."

Assertive agreement. Acknowledge criticism you agree with. You don't need to give an explanation unless you wish to. "You're right. I did botch the Sudswell account." "Thanks for pointing out that I was smiling when I was trying to say no to that salesman. No wonder I couldn't get rid of him." "You're right, boss, I am half an hour late...my car broke down."

Clouding. When someone puts you down as a person, acknowledge something in the criticism you can agree with, and ignore the rest. *Agree in part:* "You're right. I am late with the report." *Agree in the probability:* "You may be right that I am often late." *Agree in the principle (agreeing with the logic without agreeing with the premise):* "If I were late as often as you say, it certainly would be a problem." When clouding, rephrase the critic's words so that you can honestly concur. By giving the appearance of agreeing without promising to change, you soon deplete the critic of any reasons to criticize you.

Assertive inquiry. Invite criticism to find out what is really bothering the other person. "I understand you don't like the way I chaired the meeting last night. What was it about my behavior that bothered you? What is it about me that you feel is pushy? What is it about my speaking out that bothers you?"

Prepare yourself against a number of typical blocking gambits that will be used to attack and derail your assertive requests. Some of the most troublesome blocking gambits include the following:

Laughing it off. Your assertion is responded to with a joke. "Only three weeks late? I've got to work on being less punctual!" Use the content-to-process shift ("Humor is getting us off the point") and/ or the broken record ("Yes, but…" "As I was saying…").

Accusing gambit. You are blamed for causing the problem. "You always cook dinner so late, I'm too tired to do the dishes afterward." Use clouding ("That may be so, but you are still breaking your commitment") or simply disagree ("Eight o'clock is not too late to do the dishes").

The beat-up. Your assertion is responded to with a personal attack. "Who are you to worry about being interrupted? You're the biggest loudmouth around here." The best strategies to use are assertive irony ("Thank you") in conjunction with the broken record or defusing ("I can see you're angry right now; let's talk about it after the meeting").

Delaying gambit. Your assertion is met with "Not now, I'm too tired" or "Another time, maybe." Use the broken record, or insist on setting a specific time when the problem can be discussed.

"Why" gambit. Every assertive statement is blocked with a series of *why* questions, such as, "Why do you feel that way… I still don't know why you don't want to go…why did you change your mind?" The best response is to use the content-to-process shift ("*Why* isn't the point. The issue is that I'm not willing to go tonight") or the broken record.

Self-pity gambit. Your assertion is met with tears and the covert message that you are being sadistic. Try to keep going through your script using assertive agreement ("I know this is causing you pain, but I need to get this resolved").

Quibbling. The other person wants to argue with you about the legitimacy of what you feel or the magnitude of the problem, and so forth. Use the content-to-process shift ("We're quibbling now and we've gotten off the main concern") with the assertion of your right to feel the way you do.

Threats. You are threatened with statements such as "If you keep harping at me like this, you're going to need another boyfriend." Use assertive inquiry ("What is it about my requests that bothers you?") as well as content-to-process shift ("This seems to be a threat") or defusing.

Denial. You are told, "I didn't do that" or "You've really misinterpreted me." Assert what you have observed and experienced, and use clouding ("It may seem that way to you, but I've observed…").

As an exercise, write out at least one example from your life for each type of manipulation listed above. Make up or borrow examples if you need to. For each example of manipulation, write an assertive response to it.

Then allow yourself to imagine or role-play with a friend the worst possible response that could be made to your scripts for change that you are most reluctant to express in real life. Become desensitized to this possible nightmare response by facing it, and then prepare your countermeasures. When you are ready, follow up by expressing your script in real life.

Continue writing out, rehearsing, and expressing your scripts for change in real life on a frequent basis. In time, the writing and rehearsing can be eliminated, except in the most challenging situations. Combine or use separately the other assertiveness skills you learned in this chapter. As with all learned behavior, your assertiveness skills will improve and your confidence will grow with practice.

Further Reading

Alberti, R. E., and M. Emmons. 2008. *Your Perfect Right*. 9th ed. San Luis Obispo, CA: Impact Publishers.

Bower, S., and G. Bower. 2004. *Asserting Yourself: A Practical Guide for Positive Change*. New York: Da Capo Press.

Butler, P. E. 1992. *Self-Assertion for Women*. Revised ed. New York: HarperCollins.

Gabor, D. 1994. *Speaking Your Mind in 101 Different Situations*. New York: Conversation Arts Media.

Jakubowski-Spector, P. 1973. "Facilitating the Growth of Women Through Assertiveness Training." *The Counseling Psychologist* 4 (1): 75–86.

Lazarus, A. 1966. "Behavioral Rehearsal Vs. Nondirective Therapy Vs. Advice in Effecting Behavior Change." *Behaviour Research and Therapy* 4 (3): 209–12.

McClure, J. S. 2003. *Civilized Assertiveness: Communication with a Backbone, Not a Bite*. Denver, CO: Albion Street Press.

Paterson, R. J. 2000. *The Assertiveness Workbook: How to Express Your Ideas and Stand Up for Yourself at Work and in Relationships*. Oakland, CA: New Harbinger Publications.

Phelps, S., and N. Austin. 2002. *The Assertive Woman*. San Luis Obispo, CA: Impact Publishers.

Salter, A. 1949/2002. *Conditioned Reflex Therapy: The Classic Book on Assertiveness That Began Behavior Therapy*. Gretna, LA: Selfhelpbook.com (A Division of the Wellness Institute, Inc.).

Smith, M. J. 2011. *When I Say No, I Feel Guilty*. Reissue ed. New York: Bantam Books.

Wolpe, J. 1958. *Psychotherapy by Reciprocal Inhibition*. Palo Alto, CA: Stanford University Press.

CHAPTER 18

Work-Stress Management

In this chapter you will learn to:

- Identify how you currently respond to work stress
- Set goals to take control of your stress at work
- Counter stressful thinking about your work
- Negotiate when in conflict
- Pace and balance yourself

Background

The classic symptoms of work burnout include pessimism, increased dissatisfaction, absenteeism, and inefficiency at the job. While you may not be on the verge of work burnout, you may be one of the growing majority of Americans who report that their work causes them stress. Job stress accounts for a tremendous amount of personal misery and billions of dollars lost annually in productivity, wages, and medical bills. Americans are waking up to the fact that work-stress management makes personal and financial sense.

What Causes Work Burnout?

Every job includes some built-in difficulties that the worker is paid to adjust to. Job difficulties alone do not cause burnout. Rather, it is the worker's lack of control over the work situation that leads to uncertainty, frustration, reduced motivation, fatigue, reduced productivity, and eventually burnout. Here are some other factors that can lead to work burnout:

- Chronic work overload

- Unfair treatment

- Impossible expectations coming from your boss

- Unsupportive or hostile coworkers

- Inadequate training

- Lack of recognition or rewards

- Conflicting values with your company, boss, or coworkers

- Unpleasant work environment

- Lack of clear direction about priorities

Even minor factors beyond your control can have a stressful impact. Consider the many unexpected interruptions in the course of your workday: special meetings, email, messages, phone calls, people dropping in, and equipment breakdowns. Think about having to go through authorized channels and dealing with bureaucratic red tape. Think about the faulty air-conditioning system or the constant din of machines, elevator music, and voices. It's also likely that your daily commute adds to your accumulated stress for the day as well.

It is a common error to associate only excessive stress with lowered productivity. *Stress underload* occurs when a job is too easy or is insufficiently challenging. As early as 1908, Robert Yerkes and John Dodson pointed out that the symptoms of stress underload are quite similar to those of stress overload: reduced efficiency, irritability, a sense of time pressure, diminished motivation, poor judgment, and accidents. We all have a unique *performance zone* within which we experience manageable stress that stimulates our energy, motivation, decision making, and productivity.

Burnout is not caused simply by too much stress in your job. If your job made no demands on you, you would be bored. Job-stress management, like stress management in general, involves finding the right types and amounts of challenge to stimulate your interest and performance without overloading you. It also requires managing those areas of your job that are inevitably distressing. Finally, it includes balancing leisure and work-related activities so that they complement one another. Work-stress management is a dynamic process over which you can exercise personal control.

Symptom-Relief Effectiveness

Work-stress management is effective in increasing your sense of control in the workplace. Increased feelings of personal control can improve job-related symptoms of guilt, irritability, depression, anxiety, and low self-esteem. Job-stress management can also reduce job-related psychosomatic symptoms, such as insomnia, fatigue, upset stomach, headaches, eating disorders, and lowered immunity to infection.

Time to Master

Over the next few days, you will identify how you currently respond to your specific work stressors, and then you can set a few goals for change. Learning how to respond more effectively to job stress will take at least a month. The habits of effective work-stress management may take two to six months to integrate into your daily life.

Five Steps Toward Managing Your Work Stress

Step 1: Identify How You Respond to Your Specific Work Stressors

What are your specific work stressors and how do you tend to respond to them? Over the next few days, observe how you respond to both big and little stresses at work. Also, reflect on your recent experiences at work to recall and identify any troublesome responses you may have had to work stressors.

You can use the My Response to Specific Work Stressors form to list your specific stresses, write down your feelings the day the stress occurs, what you say to yourself about it, and what you do in response to it. First look at how Patty, a computer programmer, wrote down the specific stressors in her job and her responses to them in the following shorthand manner.

Patty's Response to Specific Work Stressors

Your Work Stressor	Your Feelings	Your Thoughts	Your Behavior
Programming	Bored, numb	"Nonstop programming makes Patty a dull girl."	Plodding, inefficient; eat sweets, drink coffee
Deadlines	Anxious	"I'll never make it!"	Work faster and longer, make mistakes
Meetings	Annoyed, impatient	"What a waste; I've got work to do."	Critical, resistant to suggestions
Vague supervisor	Insecure, confused, annoyed	"What does it take to please this jerk?"	Guess what he wants, complain
Chatty coworker	Angry	"Why does he keep interrupting me? He's so inconsiderate!"	Respond politely and return to my own work
Uncooperative administrative assistant	Angry, frustrated, dissatisfied	"She's lazy, slow, and utterly useless."	Refuse to talk to her
No privacy	Annoyed	"Hard to focus."	Tense my muscles; neck pain and backache
Working at a terminal	Strained, tired	"I wish I didn't have to do this."	Eyestrain, headache
Downtime	Frustrated, refreshed	"Damn, I lost everything I just wrote!"	Eat, drink coffee, socialize
No raise	Angry, frustrated	"I deserve better than this!"	Complain bitterly

Now list your specific work stressors and describe how you respond to them. Use as little or as much detail as you need.

My Response to Specific Work Stressors

Your Work Stressor	Your Feelings	Your Thoughts	Your Behavior

Now that you have written out your specific job stressors and how you typically respond to them, review your list and see whether any troublesome patterns emerge.

For example, Patty found the following patterns in her response to workplace stressors:

1. *I respond to boredom and frustration by eating too much and drinking too much coffee.*

2. *Working at a computer terminal for long periods of time and having to concentrate in spite of a lack of privacy causes me a variety of physical and emotional symptoms of stress.*

3. *I waste time because I'm not assertive enough to ask my supervisor questions, say no to my office-mate, or request administrative assistant support firmly enough.*

4. *I tend to be highly critical of myself, others, and my environment, but I rarely do anything constructive to improve my situation. I can see why I feel chronically irritated and tense at work.*

Write down any patterns you see in your responses to work stressors.

My Problematic Responses to Work Stressors

1. _____

_____

2. _____

_____

3. _____

_____

4. _____

_____

Step 2: Set Goals to Respond More Effectively to Your Work Stressors

Now that you've identified your patterns of stress in your workplace, you can begin to formulate a more effective plan for responding to any stressors that you can anticipate. Maybe you can avoid some of them altogether. Perhaps you can be better prepared for them when they happen. The name of the game is taking more control...and this is where you begin to do it.

You will probably want to make changes in one or more of the following general areas:

1. Change the external stressor (quit the job, assertively tell the boss not to overload you, take regular breaks, reorganize your time).

2. Change your thoughts (learn how to turn off work when you go home, alter your perfectionist attitude, stop assuming that you are responsible for others' problems, stop dwelling on vague worries or old injustices).

3. Change physically (relax, exercise, eat properly, get sufficient sleep).

When you are designing goals for yourself, remember the following guidelines. Remember that useful, attainable goals are:

- Specific

- Observable

- Achievable within a certain time frame

- Broken down into small intermediate steps

- Compatible with long-term goals

- Written down in simple self-contract form

- Reevaluated at specified intervals

- Rewarded when achieved

For example, Patty decided to set a new, more effective response to each of her four stress patterns as a goal. To that end, she wrote out the following self-contract.

October 10th

I, Patty Bowers, agree to change my four old patterns of responding to stress in the following ways:

Patterns 1 and 2: Rather than eating or drinking coffee when I am tired, bored, or frustrated, I will take regular breaks once an hour in which I'll either do a brief relaxation exercise or I'll get up and walk around and talk to people. I'll take advantage of flextime and go to an aerobics class three days a week and run personal errands two days a week in the middle of the day. I will eat three nutritious meals a day rather than snacking on junk food.

Pattern 3: I will enroll in a one-day workshop on assertiveness training, and I will ask my supervisor more questions until I am sure I know what he wants. I also will tell my chatty coworker not to interrupt me with small talk, other than when I get up and walk around. I will assertively ask the administrative assistant for help.

Pattern 4: I will take each one of my critical thoughts and turn it into a constructive action thought. For instance, rather than saying about meetings "What a waste, I have work to do," I could say, "Whew, a break from programming! I could do a relaxation exercise. I may learn something interesting. Also, I might contribute something to the meeting."

I will reevaluate my progress for each goal on a weekly basis. After one month, I plan to spend a weekend at a local hot springs as my reward for changing these four patterns.

Patty Bowers

Using the Self-Contract form on the next page, write out your goals to modify a few of your responses to the specific stresses in your work life.

Self-Contract

Date: _____

_____ , agree to:

1. _____

   _____

2. _____

   _____

3. _____

   _____

4. _____

   _____

I will monitor my progress every _____ (length of time).

I will reward myself with _____.

Signature: _____

Post this contract in a place where you will see it every day to remind you of what you are to do. If you like, share the contract with a friend or coworker who can encourage and support you to follow through with your plan. You can report back to that person on your progress toward each goal on a weekly basis. Remember to reward yourself when you achieve your objectives.

Step 3: Change Your Thinking

Work stress occurs, in part, because your thoughts trigger a painful emotional reaction. Here are three generic thoughts that can do you in:

1. "I've got to do (*a certain task*) (*perfectly*) (*on time*) (*so my boss will be pleased*) or (*something painful*) will happen."

2. "They're doing this to me and it's not fair."

3. "I'm trapped here."

The first thought makes you anxious, the second triggers anger, and the third generates depression. You can do something about these thoughts and the work stress they create. Right now, list the things you tell yourself about your job that fit into each of the above three categories.

Category 1:

_____

_____

_____

Category 2:

_____

_____

_____

Category 3:

_____

_____

_____

Here's how you can cope with these stress-producing thoughts:

1. Make a realistic appraisal of what exactly will happen if the task isn't finished on time, absolutely flawless, or totally pleasing to your boss. A realistic appraisal means looking at what happened to you and others in the past when tasks like this one were late, had errors, and so on. "Realistic" also means being specific. It's time to get rid of that vague sense of doom. Exactly what is your boss likely to say to you? What, if anything, is likely to happen to you?

Example: *If I don't meet Friday's deadline, it's likely that my boss will tell me to come in on the weekend to get this report done for Monday's meeting with the client. I'll have to put off going shopping with my friends. Disappointing, but I can handle that.*

Exercise: Now it's your turn. Rewrite each of your vague, catastrophic thoughts by filling in the blanks in the following sentence:

"If (*a certain task*) isn't (*perfect, on time, totally acceptable*), (*something realistic*) is likely to happen. I can handle it."

Mentally repeat this coping statement each time you catch yourself having catastrophic thoughts about vague and dire consequences. Note: If you have no idea what will happen, find out: for example, you could say, "Boss, if I'm a day late with the Crocker report, will that be a problem?"

2. Absolutely no good that can come from blaming anyone else for your work stress. Blaming maintains your sense of being stuck, helpless, and trapped. Blaming encourages you to see yourself as a victim who has no alternatives and has lost the power of choice. Blaming triggers anger and stress hormones like adrenaline that deplete your energy and, over the long run, damage your health.

    As stated in chapter 12, "Refuting Irrational Ideas," "The conditions for things or people to be otherwise don't exist.… They are what they are because of a long series of causal events.…" Rather than blaming circumstances and others, you will find it more fruitful to focus on what you can do to improve a situation.

    No one is supposed to take care of or protect you on your job. Your coworkers and supervisors are all busy taking care of and protecting themselves. This is natural: this is an inescapable fact of working life. So what can you say to yourself to stop wasting any more of your energy on blaming and anger?

Exercise: To answer this question, ask yourself, "What steps can I take to change the conditions I don't like?"

A. _____

_____

B. _____

_____

C. _____

_____

If you can't think of a way to change the conditions you don't like at work, you have two rational choices. You must either adapt to and accept the conditions or look for another job.

Exercise: If you decide to accept the current situation, fill in the blanks in the following coping statement: "_____ is acting exactly as he/she should. The conditions necessary for him/her to act this way _____ (*his/her needs and the coping strategies to meet those needs, past successes and failures, fears, attitudes toward our relationship*) all exist, and this is why he/she did (*to*) _____ (*with*) me."

4. You are not trapped. You may have difficult choices, but you aren't trapped. Right now the pain of your job seems less than the pain associated with your other available choices. Is this really true? Here's a chance to explore your options for change and compare them with the option of doing nothing.

   Exercise: What specific steps could you take to change a major stress producer at your job?

   _____

   _____

   _____

   What would you risk in attempting that change?

   _____

   _____

   _____

   What steps could you take to change jobs altogether?

   _____

   _____

   _____

   What would you risk in attempting to make that change?

   _____

   _____

   _____

What steps could you take to change your perception of a risk so that you would be willing to try to make a change?

_____

_____

_____

Typically, making a change involves acquiring additional information so that you feel more confident in your ability to cope with the challenges involved. For example, if you think that the risk in changing jobs is that you are too old, you might set as a goal asking someone your age who is employed in the type of position you want whether your age will really make a difference. Or, if you believe that you risk blowing an interview for a new position in your present company, you could set taking an interview class as a goal.

If you are not ready to do whatever is necessary to effect change, rather than saying "I'm trapped," the more accurate statement to make to yourself is "I choose to stay with the current conditions on this job because right now it seems less painful than doing (*list the steps necessary to effect change*)

_____

_____

I may choose differently in the future."

Step 4: When in Conflict, Negotiate

Whether your disagreement is with your boss regarding your salary or with your coworkers about who is supposed to make the coffee, you need to present your position and negotiate a compromise you can all live with.

Read chapter 17, "Assertiveness Training," to learn how to express your opinions, feelings, and wants as you negotiate for change. At the very least, read Step 7: Arriving at a Workable Compromise. Here is a four-step model to follow when you want to discuss a specific problem with your supervisor or coworkers with the aim of arriving at a mutually acceptable outcome. State:

1. The problem (what you perceive to be the cause of your stress)

2. How you feel about the problem

3. How it affects your productivity and motivation

4. A win-win solution (both sides of the conflict get something positive from your solution)

For example, Randy, a creative high school teacher, was refused compensation for the time he spent developing new courses. Randy told his principal, "Ever since I realized I wouldn't receive money for my course development work, my enthusiasm for teaching has deteriorated. I think my students have gained tremendous value from my new, special classes. They're now suffering as a result of my loss of motivation. It's important to me and to the school to continue creating new classes and it's important for me to be compensated in some way. Since the money isn't available, I would be satisfied to be reimbursed with time. If I could take one class period each day for an entire semester to develop my new class, that would work for me and the school." The principal's response was, "I can't spare you a class hour every day, but I can agree to give you three hours a week." Randy accepted this workable compromise.

Use the following exercise to negotiate a mutually acceptable outcome.

Exercise: Think of something you want at work that would require you to convince someone else to cooperate with you. Fill in the following blanks:

"The problem as I see it is: _____

_____.

I feel _____ about this problem.

It affects my productivity or motivation in that _____

_____.

I suggest we try this win-win solution: _____

_____."

Change the wording to fit the situation. Memorize your short script, and then look for an appropriate moment to share it with the person whose cooperation you are seeking. Remember to be open to hearing that person's point of view and look for a workable compromise that can benefit the two of you.

Step 5: Pace and Balance Yourself

Do you pace yourself at work? If you are like a sprinter, you can afford to throw everything you've got into the race. That's because at the end of a fast, short run you know you have plenty of time to recover from your intense effort. Most jobs, however, require you to be more like the marathon runner who must pace himself in order to get across the finish line in a timely manner without collapsing. Like the marathon runner, you need to maintain a certain detachment from the immediate demands of your job so that you will remember to reserve enough energy to deal with what you anticipate down the road as well as any surprises.

Here are eight tips for pacing and balancing yourself:

1. Pay attention to your natural rhythms to determine when you tend to perform optimally, and schedule your most difficult tasks for that time in your day.

2. Try to set up your day so you shift back and forth between pleasant and more difficult tasks. After finishing a tough assignment, make an effort to schedule something you enjoy.

3. Schedule periods of time into your day for work-related tasks that are pleasurable though not terribly productive. These time periods should be sacrosanct. Try to do this even when you feel rushed.

4. Take advantage of your coffee breaks and lunches to do things that will reverse the stress response. For example, go to a quiet place and do a relaxation exercise. A ten-minute brisk walk will give you as much energy as a cup of coffee. A pleasant conversation with your coworkers will release tension and may be just what you need to get a fresh perspective on a problem that is weighing you down.

5. If you are fortunate enough to have a flexible schedule, consider taking a long break in the middle of the day to do aerobic exercise or a relaxation exercise, or to run personal errands.

6. Take mini-breaks throughout your day to reduce or prevent symptoms of tension and stress. These breaks need not take more than a few minutes, and the payoff can be seen in increased mental alertness and productivity. See chapter 10, "Brief Combination Techniques," for exercises appropriate for short breaks.

7. Choose leisure activities that balance the unique stresses of your job.

If your job requires:	Consider a complementary leisure activity such as:
Much sitting or mental concentration	Aerobic exercise
Mindless repetition	Intellectually challenging hobbies and interests
A controlled environment	Hiking in nature; adventure
Boring tasks or no recognition	Competitive or achievement-oriented activities
Responding to people's demands	Solitary activities
Dealing with conflicts	Peaceful activities
Working alone	Social activities

8. Carefully plan the timing and type of vacations you take to maximize their recuperative effects.

Exercise: List at least three ways you can better pace yourself at work and create more balance in your life:

1. _____

   _____

2. _____

   _____

3. _____

   _____

Final Thoughts

It's to be expected that from time to time you will feel stressed by some aspects of your work. This chapter has shown you how you have the power to make positive changes to reduce if not eliminate that stress. Now it is up to you to use your power. In addition to the chapters on assertiveness training and refuting irrational ideas, the chapter on goal setting and time management can also help you decrease work stress.

Further Reading

Arden, J. B. 2002. *Surviving Job Stress: How to Overcome Workday Pressures.* Franklin Lakes, NJ: Career Press.

Bailey, K., and K. Leland. 2006. *Watercooler Wisdom.* Oakland, CA: New Harbinger Publications.

Dolan, S. L. 2007. *Stress, Self-Esteem, Health and Work.* London: Palgrave Macmillan.

Dunn, G. 2016. *Revivement: Having a Life After Making a Living.* Novato, CA: Having a Life Now Publishers.

Maddi, S. R., and D. M. Khoshaba. 2005. *Resilience at Work: How to Succeed No Matter What Life Throws You.* New York: Amacom Books.

Stranks, J. 2005. *Stress at Work: Management and Prevention.* Oxford, UK: Elsevier Butterworth-Heinemann Publications.

Yerkes, R. M., and J. D. Dodson. 1908. "The Relationship of Strength of Stimulus to Rapidity of Habit Formation." *Journal of Comparative Neurology and Psychology* 18 (5): 459–82.

Recording

Morgenstern, J. 2004. *Making Work Work: New Strategies for Surviving and Thriving at the Office* (Abridged Audio CD). New York: Harper Audio.

CHAPTER 19

Nutrition and Stress

In this chapter you will learn to:

- **Assess your current eating habits**
- **Eat a balanced diet to optimize health**
- **Improve your eating habits to manage stress**

Background

You would agree that eating well-balanced, nutritious meals is good for your health. Yet when under the pressure of many daily obligations or even just a single major challenge, you probably don't eat as well as you know you should. You may even skip meals and then later overeat because you are famished. Prepared foods from grocery stores, fast-food restaurants, and vending machines make it easy to eat on the run. Unfortunately, these tasty, high-calorie options often are loaded with fat, sugar, and salt. People joke that these are the three main food groups in the American diet. What is no joking matter is Americans' tendency to supersize their portions. Poor eating combined with lack of exercise contributes to our nation's high rates of health problems such as degenerative joint disease, high blood pressure, diabetes, and cardiovascular disease. Adult obesity rates have increased from 15 percent of the population in 1980 to 35 to 41 percent in recent years (CDC 2018).

You learned in chapter 1 that during acute stress, the body secretes hormones that trigger the fight-or-flight response, and nonessential physical processes, such as eating, are put on hold. During chronic stress, however, hormones such as cortisol stimulate appetite, especially for foods high in fat and sugar. If it is not immediately used as energy, this food is stored as body fat until needed in the future. If you happen to live in stressful times with frequent food scarcity, this is a real advantage. In addition, these foods do actually seem to help tamp down many of the negative effects of the stress response, hence the expression "comfort foods." Unfortunately, in a society of food abundance, cravings for your favorite comfort foods may lead to stress-induced overeating, which adds to the risk of unwanted weight gain along with other health problems (Harvard Health Publishing 2018).

Preparing and eating well-balanced nutritious meals will help counter unhealthy eating patterns during times of stress. In addition to being an opportunity to nourish your body, mealtime can be an opportunity to relax alone or with others. Consider the big picture: people of all cultures celebrate holidays and life passages, preparing and sharing delicious food. Mealtime can be an integral part of social bonding and give life joy and meaning. These social connections provide invaluable support and make coping with stressful problems more bearable.

This chapter provides guidelines for a healthy diet that you can use to set your own goals for improving your eating habits in good times and bad. You don't have to be a gourmet chef to make and enjoy nutritious, well-balanced meals.

Symptom-Relief Effectiveness

A healthy body responds to the inevitable stresses of life better than an unhealthy one, and good nutrition is an essential building block of good health. Eating well can help prevent or control high blood pressure, heart disease, indigestion, constipation, hypoglycemia, diabetes, and obesity. Good eating habits may also reduce irritability, PMS, headaches, and fatigue.

Time to Master

Plan to keep a food diary for three days. Instructions for how to keep a daily food diary appear later in the chapter. After reading this chapter's guidelines for healthy eating, compare them with your own eating habits and then decide what changes you want to make in your diet. You can begin to apply the recommendations in this chapter in a matter of hours. To make lasting changes in your diet, plan on gradually introducing a few changes at a time that you can stick with for a minimum of one month.

Twelve Steps to Healthy Eating

These twelve steps to healthy eating will help you feel better today and stay healthy for tomorrow. They are drawn from the *2015–2020 Dietary Guidelines for Americans* published jointly by the US Department of Health and Human Services (HHS) and the US Department of Agriculture (USDA) (2015). These guidelines provide authoritative advice on how good dietary habits can promote health and reduce risk for major chronic diseases, and offer tips on healthful food preparation and healthy eating.

The twelve steps include making smart choices from all food groups, finding the right balance between eating and physical activity, eating frequent calm meals, planning ahead, maximizing the nutritional value of your calories, cutting back on fats and sugar, limiting sodium, attaining or maintaining your ideal weight, limiting caffeine and alcohol, and taking vitamins.

The USDA has replaced its food pyramid guidelines with MyPlate. The image of a place setting with plate and the glass shows healthy portions of the five food groups in a balanced meal (USDA 2018). Proteins take up about one-fourth of the plate. Vegetables and fruits take up approximately half of the plate. Grains complete the plate, and a serving of dairy (milk) is part of the meal. How close is your typical meal to MyPlate?

1. Make Smart Food Choices by Eating a Variety of Foods

It is important not to limit yourself to only a few of your favorite foods in each food group. You need over forty nutrients for optimum health. Unfortunately, there is no perfect food. Even milk, which provides the basis of a baby's diet, doesn't supply vitamin C or iron, which is why we include fruit and cereal among baby's first foods. Even the natural foods favored by many health-conscious people can contain naturally toxic components. For instance, potatoes contain traces of arsenic and solanine—chemicals that are safe in low doses but poisonous at high ones (Croco 1981). Varying your diet helps maximize your nutrients and minimize your exposure to any toxic substance or contaminant.

You might be wondering how you can eat a wide variety of foods from the five food groups and not consume more calories than you need to maintain your weight. The answer is to pay attention to the serving size of what you eat and drink. A serving is a measured amount of food. The 2015 *Dietary Guidelines* recommend the number and size of servings of foods you choose within each food group. The following recommendations are for a person with a daily diet of 2,000 calories. They include suggestions for maximizing the nutritional value of the food choices you make.

Make half your grains whole. Eat six servings of grains daily, including bread, rice, cereal, and pasta products, the proverbial staff of life. At least three of these choices should be whole grains, such as whole grain breads or pasta, to add fiber to your diet. Enriched grain products restore the known nutrients that may be removed by milling. When you do buy refined foods, be sure they are enriched to restore the B vitamins and iron lost in milling. Six servings may seem like a lot, but it really isn't. Many people eat two servings of cereal at breakfast. A sandwich provides at least two servings of bread, and a plate of spaghetti easily provides two servings of pasta. A slice of bread or half a cup of rice, cereal, or pasta is a serving.

Vary your veggies. Aim for a total of 2½ cups or more of veggies daily. Be sure to select vegetables of different colors to obtain all the nutrients and antioxidants required for optimum health. It is recommended to eat at least 3 cups of dark green veggies, 2 cups of orange veggies, and 3 cups of starchy veggies weekly.

Focus on fruits. Eat fresh fruits rather than drinking fruit juice. Try for a total of 2 cups daily; for example, one small banana, one large orange, and six to eight dried apricot halves. Dried fruit makes an easy, nutritious snack; remember that dried fruit has the same calories as the fruit had before it was dried, so if you would eat one fresh pear, eat no more than two dried pear halves.

Concentrate on calcium-rich foods. Consume the equivalent of 3 cups of low-fat or fat-free milk every day. Substitute 1 ounce of cheese or a half-cup cottage cheese or a cup of yogurt for a glass of milk. Fortified soy beverages can serve as a calcium source.

Go lean with protein. Consume 5 to 6 ounces of protein daily. Read labels and choose meat items that have less than 3 grams of fat per serving. Using beans and legumes liberally in your diet will help keep your protein intake up and your fat content down. A half cup of cooked beans, lentils, or soy products is the equivalent of 1 ounce of meat. Choose fish for the omega-3 fatty acids that help control your low-density lipoprotein (LDL) cholesterol. Be aware that some fish have more fat than lean red meat and that red meat contains the iron that most women need. Bake, broil, or barbecue to reduce fat. Remove the skin from chicken before cooking, since just the skin on one chicken breast has 5 grams of fat. The restriction on eggs was relaxed in 2015 because it has been determined that dietary cholesterol does not have a direct relationship to blood cholesterol. Eggs provide inexpensive, high-quality protein, omega-3 fats, and many vitamins and iron. They are good snacks and are very portable. Up to seven eggs weekly are allowed on a healthy diet. One egg equals 1 ounce of protein.

Oils and fats. Aim for a maximum of 6 teaspoons of fat daily; most should be monounsaturated fats and oils. Get a measuring teaspoon out of the drawer and visualize how much a teaspoon of fat is. Monounsaturated oils include olives and olive oil and avocado, peanut, and canola oil. Minimize trans fats and saturated fats like coconut oil and butter. Saturated fats should not exceed 22 grams daily. Check your labels to learn the fat content of products.

Discretionary calories. These are your luxury food choices that add fat and sugar. Less than 10 percent of your calories should come from added sugars. For a 2,000-calorie diet, this is 200 calories. An oatmeal cookie might be a good choice.

Eating grains, fruits, and veggies that provide starch improves your sense of well-being. You'll notice that complex carbohydrates and fiber make meals more filling and satisfying. Carbohydrates can also function as edible tranquilizers because they contain tryptophan, an amino acid that stimulates the production of serotonin in the brain. Serotonin has a calming effect that eases tension and may cause drowsiness. Is this the explanation for that happy full feeling that a big spaghetti dinner seems to create? Eating a variety of fresh fruits and vegetables is also good for your peace of mind, since these power foods contain vitamins, minerals, and fiber and may lower the risk of health problems, including type 2 diabetes, some types of cancer, heart disease, high blood pressure, kidney stones, bone loss, and eye and digestive problems (USDA 2016; Harvard School of Public Health 2018).

Evidence continues to build that dietary fiber (including cellulose, gums, pectin, and lignin) is an essential component of a healthy diet. Fiber helps prevent or reduce constipation by increasing stool bulk and decreasing stool transit time. Shorter transit time reduces the risk of colon cancer and diverticulitis. The fiber in whole grains helps control blood sugar by slowing carbohydrate release into the bloodstream. Fiber decreases blood lipids by binding with the lipids and removing them from the body

Although the recommended intake of dietary fiber is 25 to 40 grams daily, the average American consumes only 5 to 10 grams. For most of us, fresh fruits and vegetables, whole grains, and legumes are the chief sources of fiber in our diets. You can supplement your fiber intake by eating more legumes and bran products or by adding bran to homemade foods. Plan to increase your fiber intake gradually, as rapid increases can lead to bloating and flatulence.

Dietary Fiber in Common Foods

Food Group	Dietary Fiber Content
Legumes	2.6–8.8 grams per serving
Bran cereals	2.5–6.5 grams per serving
Fruits and vegetables	2.8–5.0 grams per serving
Grains and starches	1.0–3.3 grams per ounce
Nuts	5.0–9.5 grams per serving

Compiled by author from several sources.

2. Balance Food and Activity

To feel good and stay healthy, it is important to combine healthy eating with regular exercise. Moderate aerobic activity five days a week provides substantial health benefits, and adults should exercise at least two hours and thirty minutes per week (Mayo Clinic 2018a). Chapter 20 discusses the value of exercise and how to create an exercise program you can stick with over time. The number of daily calories you need will depend upon how active you are; a calorie is simply a unit that measures the energy content of food. To maintain your current weight, you need to burn as many calories as you take in. An average woman needs 2,000 calories a day to maintain her weight, while an average man needs 2,500 calories (Gunnars 2018b). You can calculate how many calories a day you personally need to maintain your current weight or reach a healthy weight over time at www.choosemyplate.gov/myplateplan. It will also give you daily-recommended amounts for each food group, based on your sex, age range, activity level, and daily calorie level.

Go to www.choosemyplate.gov/body-weightplanner if you are interested in reaching a healthy weight in a specific amount of time and would like to calculate your recommended daily calorie level, combined with your weekly exercise commitment, to attain your goal. Keep in mind that all these numbers are just estimates, and you will need to adjust your diet and exercise program depending on your personal preferences, metabolism, and health concerns.

Here is a convenient summary of the number of daily servings of food in each food group recommended in the 2015 *Dietary Guidelines*. Look across the chart to find your recommended daily calorie level, and then look down from that number for your daily servings of food in each food group.

Healthy Portions Checklist

Daily Amount of Food from Each Food Group									
Food Plan Calories/ Day	1,200	1,400	1,600	1,800	2,000	2,200	2,400	2,600	2,800
Fruits	1 cup	1.5 cups	1.5 cups	1.5 cups	2 cups	2 cups	2 cups	2 cups	2.5 cups
Veggies	1.5 cups	1.5 cups	2 cups	2.5 cups	2.5 cups	3 cups	3 cups	3.5 cups	3.5 cups
Grains	2 cups	2.5 cups	2.5 cups	3 cups	3 cups	3.5 cups	4 cups	4.5 cups	5 cups
Meat/poultry/ eggs/soy/nuts/ seeds	3 ounces	4 ounces	5 ounces	5 ounces	5.5 ounces	6 ounces	6.5 ounces	6.5 ounces	7 ounces
Milk/dairy	2.5 cups	2.5 cups	3 cups	3 cups	3 cups	3 cups	3 cups	3 cups	3 cups
Oils	4 tsp.	4 tsp.	5 tsp.	5 tsp.	6 tsp.	6 tsp.	7 tsp.	8 tsp.	8 tsp.
Discretionary	100	110	130	170	270	280	350	380	400

3. Eat Frequent, Calm Meals

Our fast-paced society encourages eating on the run. To counter stress, take time out to relax while you prepare and eat your meals and snacks. Blood sugar is like gasoline for a car; we all know a car won't run if its fuel tank is empty. Eating three to five small meals a day helps maintain an even blood-sugar level.

At work, find a comfortable place away from your workstation to sit and relax with your meal or snack. If possible, take some time alone to relax and reflect during your breaks. Learn to savor the flavors, textures, and colors of your food.

4. Create a Meal Plan for the Week

Map your meals with a weekly menu and grocery list to save time and ensure that you have the ingredients for simple meals in your cupboard and refrigerator. When you cook, prepare enough for additional meals or snacks. It's cheaper, quicker, easier, and healthier to reheat something in the microwave than to run out to buy a fast-food meal.

Love your leftovers. For lunch at work, take some healthy leftovers or bring a sandwich on whole wheat bread. Drink water, a sugar-free beverage, or a serving of low-fat milk, and take a piece of fruit for dessert. This is cheaper and healthier than eating at the deli.

When running errands, chauffeuring, or commuting, take along some sliced-up fruit, baby carrots, string cheese, or raw almonds.

If you don't have time to prepare a meal from scratch, check out the many tasty nutritious convenience foods now available in your grocery store's fresh and frozen food sections and read the ingredients. Ready-roasted chicken from the grocery can also provide the basis of several meals. You can save time and focus on good nutrition if you use some creativity in planning and preparing your meals. These activities will give you a sense of control and help decrease stress.

5. Maximize the Nutrition in Your Calories and Limit Sugar

It's important to choose a wide variety of nutritionally rich foods each day; choose foods that are packed with vitamins, minerals, fiber, and other micronutrients. Pick fresh fruits, whole grains, and low-fat dairy products. Look at nutrition labels to make your calories count. Any food item with over 400 calories per serving is too high in calories.

Sugars contribute many calories without nutrients to your diet, so use foods low in added sugars. Sugars include sucrose, glucose, fructose, high-fructose corn syrup, corn syrup, honey, and maple syrup. Americans have a sweet tooth. If you've been abroad, you've probably noticed that American desserts tend to be much sweeter than desserts from other parts of the world. Including table sugar, sugar in soft drinks, canned foods, baked goods, and other sweets, the average American now eats 19.5 teaspoons of sugar daily. Excessive sugar intake is common. It's been linked with various lifestyle diseases, including obesity, type 2 diabetes and prediabetes, and heart disease (Gunnars 2018a).

As children, we were given sweets to comfort us. As adults, when we are stressed, we still reach for cookies, candy, or sweets. Women are more likely to seek solace in sweets than men are. Scientists think that sweets trigger the release of endorphins, the natural opiates that create euphoric feelings. Although sugar may provide a temporary high, it also stimulates the pancreas to secrete insulin to process the sugar. The pancreas sometimes overreacts and secretes excess insulin. The result can be hypoglycemia, a condition characterized by dizziness, irritability, nausea, and hunger pangs that may, in turn, prompt a craving for another sweet treat. Cravings for sweets are best satisfied with a piece of fruit. Fruit provides the complex sugars, fiber, and vitamins that sugary foods lack.

Clues for cutting sugar:

- Use less sugar, raw sugar, honey, and corn or maple syrup.

- Eat fewer foods that contain sugar, such as candy, cookies, and soft drinks.

- Select fresh fruit or fruits canned in juice or light syrup rather than heavy syrup.

- Avoid processed foods with sucrose, glucose, maltose, dextrose, lactose, or fructose listed as first ingredients.

6. Cut Back on Fats

Despite all the bad press that fat has received, the average American ingests significantly more total calories from fat (37 to 42 percent) than the 20 to 30 percent or less recommended by the 2015 *Dietary Guidelines*. We talk about cutting fat, but when we get hungry, we still reach for our high-fat favorites, despite the presence of so many alternatives. The food industry has come up with dozens of new lower-fat snack and cookie products to help you make the change, but fruit or vegetable sticks are the best low-fat snacks. Bookstores, magazines, and websites are full of low-fat recipes that offer menus full of tasty and creative dishes. Fat-free salad dressings or flavored vinegars provide other ways to reduce the fat in your diet. Even those people with no time to cook can fall back on "lean" or "healthy" frozen entree products. Be sure to check the label and select items with 3 grams or fewer of fat per serving.

There are three kinds of fat. Saturated fat is solid at room temperature and is usually of animal origin. Examples are visible meat fat, chicken skin, and butter. Crisco is an example of a trans fat, or an oil that has been highly saturated, or hydrogenated. Polyunsaturated fats, like corn and safflower oil, remain liquid even when refrigerated. Monounsaturated fat is liquid at room temperature but solidifies when chilled. Monounsaturated oils, such as canola and olive oil, are now recommended over polyunsaturated oils. Although the exact relation of fats to hypertension and heart disease is still controversial, the most widely accepted theory is that saturated and trans fats contribute to heart disease and strokes by elevating the body's cholesterol level. The 2015 *Dietary Guidelines* recommend a saturated fat intake under 10 percent total calories, general fat intake of 20 to 35 percent of total calories, or 400 to 700 fat and oil calories daily in a 2,000 calorie diet.

Most fat creeps into our diet via fried foods, baked goods, snack foods, and other processed foods. Limiting these foods is the best way to cut fat and cut calories too. Potato chips and tortilla chips have 7 to 10 grams of fat per serving, and it is hard to stop at one serving! Crackers have about 5 grams of fat per serving. Pretzels usually have no fat. Baked goods, especially with frosting, have high fat content. Fried foods, of course, contribute fat to the diet. Kentucky Fried Chicken's Original Recipe chicken breast has 28 grams of fat and 6 grams of saturated fat.

Dietary products to reduce or modify fat intake are widely available on the market, but there are yet no long-term studies of their impact on health. Molly McButter is a low-calorie butter substitute. Products containing omega-3 fats are available to assist in reducing triglyceride and cholesterol levels. Fat replacers like Olestra are chemically altered so that they pass through the body unabsorbed and will take some fat-soluble vitamins along with them.

How Do You Score on Fat Intake?

Answer the following questions by circling the number in the column that best describes how often you select or limit the foods listed on the scorecard. Add up the numbers you circled for your total score.

Your Fat Score: Do You...?	Rarely	Often	Always
Choose lean meat, chicken, or fish?	1	5	10
Eat high-fat meats like bacon, lunch meats, or sausage?	10	5	1
Eat fish twice weekly?	1	5	10
Read labels and select foods with less than 3 grams of fat per serving?	1	5	10
Choose low-fat or nonfat dairy products?	1	5	10
Limit fried foods?	1	5	10
Choose donuts, croissants, or sweet rolls for breakfast?	10	5	1
Choose reduced-fat or fat-free products or limit fats?	1	5	10
Use olive oil or canola oil often?	1	5	10
Balance a high-fat dinner with a low-fat breakfast and lunch?	1	5	10

Insert your fat score: _____

Scoring: If you scored 10 to 59 points, you can do better. At 60 to 79 points, you're on your way. If you scored over 80 points, keep up the good work!

7. Reduce Your Sodium Intake

Although sodium is an essential mineral, most adults in the United States ingest more than the recommended sodium requirement. The USDA's dietary reference intake (DRI) for recommended daily sodium intake is 1,300 to 1,500 milligrams (mg) for adults or less than one teaspoon of salt a day. One teaspoon of salt contains 2,300 mg of sodium. Generally, adult men average more salt than 4,200 mg daily and women average 3,300 mg daily (DRI). Sodium regulates body fluids, maintains pH balance, and controls nerve and muscle activities.

Our major sodium sources are table salt (composed of 40 percent sodium and 60 percent chloride) and processed foods. Sodium is a natural component of milk, cheese, meats, and bread. Check the label, and if any food serving has more than 500 mg of sodium, the salt content is too high, since it contributes more than 20 percent of your daily total. If hypertension runs in your family, you may want to restrict sodium with the DASH (Dietary Approaches to Stop Hypertension) plan of eating, which is recommended in the 2015 *Dietary Guidelines*. Information about this plan is available on the Internet or at your bookstore. If you have severe hypertension, the *Dietary Guidelines* suggest restricting sodium to 1,500 mg daily. Be sure to discuss this with your doctor.

A high intake of sodium correlates with high blood pressure and increased risk of stroke. Since stress also aggravates these conditions, you will be wise to reduce your salt intake. Salt also increases edema, an excess accumulation of fluid that adds to the stress of premenstrual syndrome. High potassium intake (lots of fruits and vegetables) counteracts some of the effects of sodium on blood pressure.

Tips for shaking the salt habit:

- Avoid salty snacks like chips, pretzels, and nuts.

- Limit your intake of salty condiments like soy sauce, pickles, and cheese.

- Restrict your use of cured meats, sausages, and bacon.

- Savor food with less salt by substituting spices and herbs.

- Do not cook with salt, and add little or no salt at the table.

- Read labels carefully. Avoid foods with salt or sodium listed in the first three to four ingredients.

8. Know Your Body Mass Index

The body mass index (BMI) is now a frequently used measure to assess body weight. BMI is a number based on a weight-height ratio that indicates your weight-related health risks. It doesn't measure body fat or take gender or age into consideration. A BMI of 18.5 to 24.9 indicates a low risk for weight-related problems. A BMI of 25 to 29.9 indicates some risk for weight-related health problems, and a BMI of over 30 indicates a significant risk for weight-related health problems. You can calculate your BMI easily at http://choosemyplate.gov/tools-BMI.

Another way to assess your health risk is waist measurement. If your BMI indicates a health risk and your waist is over 35 inches for women or more than 40 inches for men, your health risks increase as your waist size increases (HHS 2018; Mayo Clinic 2018b). Research also indicates that people with apple-shaped bodies have more health risk factors than those with pear-shaped bodies, who carry their weight on their hips and thighs (American Heart Association News 2018).

9. Maintain a Healthy Weight

Although there are thousands of weight-reduction diets, the best weight-control strategy is a lifelong sensible eating plan. Current research indicates that yo-yo dieting damages health and makes each successive attempt to lose weight even harder.

Diets usually don't work. After all, diets represent food deprivation, which is emotionally difficult for most of us. In addition, your body interprets the diet regime as a famine, and it reduces your overall metabolic rate to decrease the impact of deprivation on your body. The more rigorous the diet, the more your body will resist losing weight. For those who do achieve significant weight loss, more than 95 percent will not keep the weight off for even one year, and they end up dieting again. This sets the yo-yo spinning, and with each new diet the body lowers the energy required for maintenance a little bit more, making weight control increasingly more difficult.

It is better to be a bit overweight than to diet continually to lose the same ten pounds repeatedly. The simple math is that you must expend the same number of calories you eat to avoid gaining weight. The ideal combination for weight loss is to eat a little less and exercise a little more. It is also possible to eat the same quantity of food, or even more, if you cut the fat content of your food.

The best approach to weight control is to reduce your daily food intake by 100 calories and to burn 100 more calories a day by increasing your exercise. This means that by cutting out one slice of bread a day and walking one mile a day more than you do now, you will be twenty pounds lighter a year from now!

Diets are just a temporary fix; weight control is a lifelong lifestyle issue. Dealing with this issue means making a commitment to low-fat cooking methods; to choosing low-calorie, low-fat foods consistently; and to being satisfied with smaller portions.

A program that provides good nutrition education and realistic exercise goals can help you make a lifelong commitment. For example, Weight Watchers, one of the most reputable programs, advocates eating lots of vegetables, cutting down on fat, and increasing exercise. It also offers behavior modification programs and support. There are Weight Watchers chapters in most cities. Other organizations that provide educational and support programs include Overeaters Anonymous, the YMCA and YWCA, as well as many health-insurance programs, local colleges, and community centers.

Good weight-control programs emphasize behavioral changes such as the following:

- Eat slowly. Take small bites and truly enjoy the color, taste, and texture of your food. After you've finished eating a meal, remember that it takes twenty minutes for the hypothalamus—the area in the brain that governs appetite and hunger—to register that you are full and to provide that feedback to your brain.

- Eat mindfully. Don't read or watch TV while eating. Enjoy eating by being aware of flavors, colors, and portion size.

- Eat regularly. People who eat three to five small meals daily are more likely to control their appetite and their weight successfully. This may be because they do not get excessively hungry and overeat. People who eat breakfast consume fewer calories, maintain healthier weights, and have reduced risk of heart disease. Studies also indicate that people who eat a healthy breakfast consume fewer total calories daily (Duyff 2012).

- Control portion size. Portions are generally a half cup. You can eat anything you want so long as the portion fits in a four-ounce Pyrex custard cup.

- Don't eat when you're bored. Substitute a different pleasurable activity, such as taking a walk, calling a friend, or engaging in a hobby.

- Don't eat when you're angry. Write a letter to the person you're angry with (but don't send it) or go jogging or do some gardening. If you must bite down on something, make sure that something is a carrot or sugarless gum.

- Don't eat when you're tired. Go to bed or take a hot bath. You may be surprised to find that a walk or a bike ride may even reenergize you.

- Don't eat when you're anxious or depressed. Engage in physical activity, go to a movie, talk to a friend, or find a way to deal with the issues contributing to the anxiety or depression.

10. Consider Your Caffeine Intake

Americans love the boost they get from the caffeine in their coffee, tea, chocolate, and colas. Some medications are also high in caffeine. Unfortunately, caffeine can contribute to irritability, nervousness, sleep difficulties, and gastrointestinal distress. Caffeine stays in your system for six hours or longer, so if you are having any of these problems, consider limiting your use of it, not drinking it after lunch, or discontinuing it altogether.

If you drink regular coffee—that is, not decaffeinated—a daily limit of 400 mg of caffeine, or four cups of coffee, is now the recommended limit in the 2015 *Dietary Guidelines*. Caffeine limits have been raised in the last few years, but caffeine may still give you the jitters or make you irritable. If not, enjoy your coffee, but not the super mochachino lattes that have a lot of sugar and fat in them. Recent findings are that coffee has lots of antioxidants and may protect against diabetes and Parkinson's disease (Shmerling 2017). Moderation in coffee and caffeine intake is advisable, as risks or any side effects are lower with moderation.

Caffeine Content of Beverages and Chocolate

Beverage or Chocolate	Serving Size	Caffeine Content
Regular coffee, brewed	8 ounces	80–135 mg, average 110 mg
Decaffeinated coffee, brewed	8 ounces	5–10 mg
Instant coffee	8 ounces	65–100 mg
Black tea, brewed	8 ounces	40–120 mg
Instant tea	8 ounces	15 mg
Green tea	12–16 ounces	15–30 mg
Canned iced tea	12 ounces	9–50 mg
Snapple iced teas	12 ounces	42 mg
Cola drinks	8 ounces	35–55 mg
Hot chocolate	8 ounces	5–15 mg
Dark chocolate candy	1 ounces	5–35 mg
Milk chocolate candy	1 ounces	5–10 mg

Compiled by author from multiple sources. Brewed beverages vary considerably.

11. Drink Alcohol in Moderation or Not at All

Although some research indicates that a drink a day may increase longevity, reliance on alcohol to deal with daily life is a dangerous practice. Alcoholic beverages are high in calories and low in nutrients. Excess alcohol depletes B vitamins, alters blood sugar, elevates blood pressure, and disrupts relationships. If you drink, limit yourself to one drink if you are a woman and two drinks if you are a man.

12. Take a Daily Multivitamin

In the early 1990s, the Food and Nutrition Board of the National Academy of Sciences undertook the task of revising recommended dietary allowances (RDAs), and the dietary reference intakes (DRIs) were born. DRIs include recommended dietary allowances, the adequate intake (AI), and the tolerable upper intake level (UL). DRIs are daily nutrient recommendations based on age and gender and are set at levels to meet the needs of healthy individuals. The recommendations include allowances for individual variation. You will also see daily values (DV) on vitamin and nutrition labels, which are based on the RDA.

Because we do not all eat according to the recommendations every day, a multivitamin tablet may serve as an insurance policy. However, taking vitamins is not a substitute for eating well. There are undoubtedly compounds in foods that we have not yet identified that are nutritionally important adjuncts to the proper functioning of vitamins and minerals in metabolism.

Vitamins and minerals are necessary in small amounts, and are required for metabolic processes. Vitamins A, E, and C are antioxidants, and taking these vitamins as supplements may be protective against some cancers, though this benefit has not yet been proven (National Cancer Institute 2017). Vitamins marketed as "stress tabs" or "stress formulations" are meant for physical stress, not psychological stress. Note that more is not better when supplementing vitamins and minerals.

Fat-soluble vitamins may become toxic because they accumulate in the liver. New evidence indicates that an overdose of water-soluble vitamins may also be toxic. Vitamin and mineral function is interrelated: vitamin C enhances iron absorption; vitamin D, calcium, and phosphorus work together in bone metabolism; and B vitamins are necessary for burning glucose as a fuel for the body. Because vitamins and minerals are interrelated, increasing intake of one often causes an imbalance somewhere else. Supplements should not exceed the tolerable upper intake level (UL) for each element, due to the danger of toxicity.

Dietary Reference Intakes (DRIs) (Recommended for Individuals)

	Men		Women	
Age	31–50	51+	31–50	51+
Fat-Soluble Vitamins				
Vitamin A (µg /d)*	**900**	900	700	700
Vitamin D (µg /d)	15	15	15	15
Vitamin E (µg TE/d)	**15**	15	15	15
Vitamin K (µg/d)	120	120	90	90
Water-Soluble Vitamins				
Vitamin C (mg/d)	90	90	75	75
Thiamine (mg/d)	1.2	1.2	1.1	1.1
Riboflavin (mg/d)	1.3	1.3	1.1	1.1
Niacin (mg/d)	16	16	14	14
Folate (µg/d)	400	400	400	400
Vitamin B_{12} (µg/d)	2.4	2.4	2.4	2.4
Minerals				
Calcium (mg/d)	1000	1000	1000	1200
Copper (µg/d)	900	900	900	900
Iodine (µg/d)	150	150	150	150
Iron (mg/d)	8	8	18	8
Magnesium (mg/d)	420	420	320	320
Phosphorus (mg/d)	700	700	700	700
Selenium (µg/d)	55	55	55	55
Zinc (mg/d)	11	11	8	8

*(µg/d) = micrograms a day; bold type = RDA, regular type = AI

Compiled by author from several DRI charts (National Academy of Sciences 2018).

Self-Assessment

Start with a Daily Food Diary

If you are interested in making significant changes in your eating habits, it will be worth your while to keep a record of everything you eat and drink for the next three days. By noting the sizes of portions, you will discover exactly how much you neglect certain food groups and overindulge in others. You will be amazed to see how sugars and fats sneak into your diet. Make a note if you see any important connections between the circumstances in which you eat and drink, your feelings, and your diet. You can then compare your food diary records with the guidelines in this chapter and create a plan for a more nutritionally balanced diet. You may want to repeat this exercise periodically to measure your progress.

Before you start, look at Sharon's food diary sample. Sharon is a five-foot-seven, forty-year-old paralegal who is moderately active and weighs 170 pounds. Notice that in addition to writing down everything that she ate, she noted the setting in which she ate and how she felt while she was eating.

Refer to Sharon's diary and the Healthy Portions Checklist to fill in the food group servings column of your Daily Food Diary. Sharon's example shows you how to count servings. Here are some specific guidelines to keep in mind:

- Note that low-fat milk counts as one milk serving and one fat serving, because nonfat milk is the recommended milk serving. Use plain or light yogurt to avoid the sugar content of yogurt with added fruit.

- Count all alcohol, cookies, cake, donuts, ice cream, or sweet rolls as discretionary and record their calories. All treats with fat or added sugar count in the discretionary group.

- Note that French fries contain at least three teaspoons of oil (equal to three servings of fat).

- Salad dressing is one fat serving for every 1 to 2 tablespoons. Use olive oil and vinegar for a healthy dressing.

Visit http://www.newharbinger.com/43348 to download the blank Daily Food Diary form, and record your food intake for at least three days. Be sure to write down where and when you eat, the setting and the people with you at the time, and your feelings. Eating is often tied to internal and external cues, and keeping track of this information may give you clues as to why you eat the way you do.

Sharon's Daily Food Diary

Meal	Food	Amount	Food Group Servings	Setting	Feelings
Breakfast	Oatmeal Low-fat milk	½ cup 1 cup	1 grains 1 milk + 1 fat	Kitchen, alone	Hungry, hurried
Snack	Crumb donut Coffee w/ sugar	1 2 cups 2 tsp.	240 calories 2 caffeine sugar: 36 calories	Coffee room	Happy, social
Lunch	Tuna sandwich on whole wheat with mayo Diet coke Apple	3 oz. 2 slices 1 tbsp. 12 oz. 5 oz.	2 meat, fish 2 grains 3 fat 1 caffeine 1 fruit	Alone at desk, working	Busy, pressured
Snack	Grapes	Medium bunch	1 fruit	Coffee room	Tense, headache
Dinner	Hamburger on whole wheat bun, lettuce & tomato, and mayo French fries	6 oz. 1 bun 2 tsp. 4 oz.	6 meat 2 grains 1 vegetable 2 fat 1 vegetable 3 fat	Home with family	Tired, grumpy
Snack	Rocky road ice cream	½ cup	250 calories	TV, alone	Tired, bored

Daily Food Diary

Meal	Food	Amount	Food Group Servings	Setting	Feelings
Breakfast					
Snack					
Lunch					
Snack					
Dinner					
Snack					

Summarizing Your Food Diary

Fill out the blank Food Diary Summary with the data you've collected. You can refer to the example of Sharon's Daily Food Diary, in which she summarized the information she collected over a three-day period. For each day that you kept your food diary, add up the total number of servings in each food group and write that number in the appropriate box on your Food Diary Summary. Average the result for each food group over the three days. Enter this daily average for each food group. At the top of the last column, fill in your food plan calories from the MyPlate calorie calculator. Then, referring to the Healthy Portions Checklist, fill in the number of healthy servings for each food group in the column. You can then compare your daily averages for each food group with the healthy portions listed in the last column.

Sharon's Food Diary Summary

Food Group Servings	Day 1	Day 2	Day 3	Daily Average	Healthy Portions for 2,000 Daily Calories
Breads and grains A serving equals 1 slice bread, ½ cup rice, cereal, or pasta.	*5 servings*	*6 servings*	*7 servings*	*6 servings*	6 servings
Fruit A serving equals ½ cup or one small apple, orange.	*1 cup*	*1 cup*	*2 cups*	*1.3 cups*	2 cups
Vegetables A serving equals ½ cup or one 4-ounce potato.	*1 cup*	*3 cups*	*2 cups*	*2 cups*	2.5 cups
Milk, cheese, yogurt A serving equals 1 cup milk or 1 ounce of hard cheese.	*1 cup*	*2 cups*	*3 cups*	*2 cups*	3 cups
Meat, poultry, fish, eggs, beans, lentils, soy products A serving of meat, fish, or chicken equals 2 to 3 ounces; 2 to 3 eggs are a serving. Four ounces of beans, lentils, or soy products equal 1 ounce of meat.	*9 ounces*	*6 ounces*	*8 ounces*	*8 ounces*	5.5 ounces
Fats and oils A serving equals 1 tsp. oil or 1 tbsp. salad dressing.	*7 tsp.*	*4 tsp.*	*6 tsp.*	*5.6 tsp.*	6 tsp.
Caffeine A serving equals 8 ounces.	*3 cups*	*2 cups*	*4 cups*	*3 cups*	0–4 servings
Discretionary calories *(includes alcohol)*	526	350	450	442	270 calories 0–1 serving

Food Diary Summary

Food Group Servings	Day 1	Day 2	Day 3	Daily Average	Healthy Portions for 2,000 Daily Calories
Breads and grains A serving equals 1 slice bread, ½ cup rice, cereal, or pasta.					6 servings
Fruit A serving equals ½ cup or one small apple, orange.					2 cups
Vegetables A serving equals ½ cup or one 4-ounce potato.					2.5 cups
Milk, cheese, yogurt A serving equals 1 cup milk or 1 ounce of hard cheese.					3 cups
Meat, poultry, fish, eggs, beans, lentils, soy products A serving of meat, fish, or chicken equals 2 to 3 ounces; 2 to 3 eggs are a serving. Four ounces of beans, lentils, or soy products equal 1 ounce of meat.					5.5 ounces
Fats and oils A serving equals 1 tsp. oil or 1 tbsp. salad dressing.					6 tsp.
Caffeine A serving equals 8 ounces.					0–4 servings
Discretionary calories (includes alcohol)					270 calories 0–1 serving

Taking Charge of Your Nutritional Well-Being

These guidelines provide a goal for daily food choices. Review your Food Diary Summary and compare your average servings per food group against healthy portions in the last column. Put a check in the margin of the groups in which you were below the recommendation. Put a star in the margin next to the groups in which you exceeded the recommendation.

After reviewing the facts presented in this chapter, is your diet more like the typical American diet or the MyPlate recommendations? Chances are that your diet overdoes it on fats and sugars and skimps on fruits, vegetables, grains, bread, and cereals.

After Sharon had reviewed her own summary, she sat down and filled out a goal-setting chart. The solutions she developed may suggest some positive steps that you can take.

Sharon's Goal-Setting Chart

Food Group	Problem	Solution
Fruit	A little short of goal	Eat fruit instead of ice cream at night.
Vegetables	I hate veggies, so I did not meet 3-cup goal, and I did not choose any green or brightly colored veggies.	Eat more salads and add one new veggie each month.
Meat, fish, eggs	Portions too large	Weigh or measure portions for one week.
Caffeine	Caffeine sensitivity, sometimes jittery	Switch to herbal teas, or walk during breaks to reduce jitters
Discretionary calories	Too many goodies	Eat fruit or light yogurt at morning break.

It's time to develop your own positive eating goals. Go back to your Daily Food Diary and review the settings in which you ate. Note anything about these settings that might contribute to unhealthy eating behavior. For example, it's clear from Sharon's sample diary that eating alone at her desk provided no break from work and may have made her less efficient as her tension level grew in the afternoon.

Having lunch with friends or, at least, in a different locale would have provided a change of scene. She usually takes her breaks in the coffee room, where high-fat, high-sugar snacks are a temptation. If she takes a piece of fruit or some light yogurt to the coffee room, she can still have the benefits of socializing, and will markedly improve the nutritional value of her break.

Set Your Personal Positive Eating Goals Now

What changes or improvements would you make regarding the setting in which you eat?

_____

_____

_____

Review the feelings that you recorded in your Daily Food Diary. Note any feelings that contributed to unhealthy eating behavior. For instance, looking at Sharon's food diary, you can see that she uses comfort food to try to feel better when she has negative feelings and sensations (tension, headaches, boredom, fatigue). Aerobic exercise, socializing, or a relaxation exercise might have been more effective for symptom reduction. She can also plan to have a favorite low-calorie substitute available for those times when she knows she is likely to feel down. Going to bed earlier might prevent her need to snack when she feels bored or tired at night. If an earlier bedtime led to getting up earlier in the morning, she would also have time for a less hurried breakfast or some exercise.

How do your feelings contribute to your dietary intake? What changes can you make?

_____

_____

_____

Changing your eating habits will take some time. Concentrate on no more than one or two goals at a time for a minimum of one month. When you have integrated these new eating habits into your daily life, set one or two more goals. Depending on how many habits you wish to change, you should be enjoying a healthier lifestyle in one to six months. Making too many changes at a time can be stressful, so go slowly. Note that the changes you make to your diet also need to be tasty ones; otherwise, you will feel deprived and have difficulty sticking with your plan.

Final Thoughts

You have the power to take charge of your eating habits, and taking charge will make a positive difference. Just keep the twelve guidelines in mind and gradually make changes in your food selections. Put a copy of MyPlate on the refrigerator as a reminder, and keep it in mind when you shop. Check online for new low-fat recipes that focus on fruits and vegetables. Browse the bookstore for a new healthy recipe book. If you need a personalized nutrition plan, consult a registered dietitian at your local medical clinic or look online for a local resource. If you have questions about nutrition, the American Academy of Nutrition and Dietetics website is a great place to start.

Food is a necessity and a pleasure in life, so make positive, healthy choices!

Further Reading

American Heart Association News. 2018. "Waist Size Predicts Heart Attacks Better than BMI, Especially in Women." *Heart Insight Magazine.* Summer. http://heartinsight.heart.org/Summer-2018/Waist-size-predicts-heart-attacks-better-than-BMI-especially-in-women/.

CDC (Centers for Disease Control). 2018. "Adult Obesity Facts." Overweight and Obesity. US Department of Health and Human Services. https://www.cdc.gov/obesity/data/adult.html.

Croco, S. 1981. "Potato Sprouts and Greening Potatoes: Potential Toxic Reaction." JAMA 245 (6): 625. Available at https://www.accessdata.fda.gov/scripts/plantox/detail.cfm?id=6537.

Duyff, R. 2012. *The American Dietetic Association Complete Food and Nutrition Guide.* 4th ed. Hoboken, NJ: John Wiley & Sons.

Editors of Cooking Light. 2013. *Cooking Light the Fresh Food Fast Cookbook: The Ultimate Collection of Top-Rated Everyday Dishes.* New York: Time Inc. Books.

Gunnars, K. 2018a. "Daily Intake of Sugar—How Much Sugar Should You Eat Per Day?" June 28. https://www.healthline.com/nutrition/how-much-sugar-per-day#section1.

———. 2018b. "How Many Calories Should You Eat Per Day to Lose Weight?" July 6. https://www.healthline.com/nutrition/how-many-calories-per-day.

Harvard Health Publishing. 2018. "Why Stress Causes People to Overeat." Harvard Mental Health Letter. First published February, 2012; updated July 18, 2018. https://www.health.harvard.edu/staying-healthy/why-stress-causes-people-to-overeat.

Harvard School of Public Health. 2018. "Vegetables and Fruits." https://www.hsph.harvard.edu/nutrition-source/what-should-you-eat/vegetables-and-fruits.

HHS (US Department of Health and Human Services). 2018. Classification of Overweight and Obesity by BMI, Waist Circumference, and Associated Disease Risks. National Heart, Lung, and Blood Institute, National Institutes of Health. https://www.nhlbi.nih.gov/health/educational/lose_wt/BMI/bmi_dis.htm.

HHS (US Department of Health and Human Services) and USDA (Department of Agriculture). 2015. *2015–2020 Dietary Guidelines for Americans.* Published jointly by the Department of Health and Human Services and the Department of Agriculture.

Mayo Clinic. 2018a. "Exercise Intensity: How to Measure It." https://www.mayoclinic.org/healthy-lifestyle /fitness/in-depth/exercise-intensity/art-20046887.

———. 2018b. "Is It True That Waist Size Can Be a Predictor of Life Expectancy?" Mayo Foundation for Medical Education and Research. June 9. https://www.mayoclinic.org/healthy-lifestyle/weight-loss /expert-answers/waist-size-and-life-expectancy/faq-20348574.

National Academy of Sciences. 2018. Dietary Reference Intakes Tables and Application. Health and Medicine Division. Updated January 16. http://nationalacademies.org/hmd/Activities/Nutrition/ SummaryDRIs/DRI-Tables.aspx.

National Cancer Institute 2017. "Antioxidants and Cancer Prevention." Reviewed February 6. https:// www.cancer.gov/about-cancer/causes-prevention/risk/diet/antioxidants-fact-sheet.

Shmerling, R. 2017. "The Latest Scoop on the Health Benefits of Coffee." *Harvard Health Blog.* September 25. https://www.health.harvard.edu/blog/the-latest-scoop-on-the-health-benefits-of-coffee-2017092512429.

USDA (Department of Agriculture). 2016. "Why Is It Important to Eat Vegetables?" Updated January 12. https://www.choosemyplate.gov/vegetables-nutrients-health.

———. 2018. "What Is MyPlate? Updated July 19. https://www.choosemyplate.gov/MyPlate.

Websites and Other Resources

American Academy of Nutrition and Dietetics: www.eatright.org

BMI Calculator: https://www.nhlbi.nih.gov/health/educational/lose_wt/BMI/bmicalc.htm

Choose MyPlate: www.choosemyplate.gov

DASH diet: www.nhlbi.nih.gov/health/public/heart/hbp/dash/new_dash.pdf

Estimated Calorie Needs Per Day Based on Physical Activity: https://www.cnpp.usda.gov/sites/default/files /usda_food_patterns/EstimatedCalorieNeedsPerDayTable.pdf

Get Your MyPlate Plan: https://www.choosemyplate.gov/MyPlatePlan

Just Enough for You: About Food Portions: https://www.niddk.nih.gov/health-information/weight-manage ment/just-enough-food-portions

Mayo Clinic: www.mayoclinic.com

Weight Watchers: (800) 651–6000

CHAPTER 20

Exercise

In this chapter you will learn:

- How exercise decreases the stress response

- How to create a well-balanced exercise program for yourself

- How to safely monitor your response to exercise

- How to motivate yourself to get started and stay committed to your exercise program

Background

The human body is designed for movement. Yet the average American sits for 9.3 hours a day in sedentary jobs with electronic devices and reports increasing symptoms of anxiety (Teychenne, Costigan, and Parker 2015). We move our bodies less than is needed to maintain good health. Research has linked several health concerns, including stress and anxiety, with sitting for long periods of time (Laskowski 2018). Less sitting and more moving contribute to overall better health. Exercise is one of the simplest and most effective means of stress management and can decrease depression as effectively as Prozac or behavioral therapy (American College of Sports Medicine 2014). Regular exercise is now routinely recommended to manage stress by major health care organizations such as the Mayo Clinic, the Cleveland Clinic, Johns Hopkins, and Kaiser Permanente. This chapter will show you how to become and remain more physically active and keep your life in better balance.

Symptom-Relief Effectiveness

Studies over the past ten years consistently support adding regular physical activity to your daily regimen for effective symptom-relief of stress and anxiety. Exercise creates chemical releases of endorphins, dopamine, and serotonin, which acts as a natural high that relieves stress (Anderson and Shivakumar 2013). Other benefits of exercise include decreased muscle tension, increased concentration, improved strength, posture, and flexibility, increased energy level, improved sleep, weight loss, and improved physical fitness and overall health.

Staying healthy involves being active, regardless of age. Regular aerobic exercise lowers sympathetic nervous system reactivity to physical and psychological stressors (Anderson and Shivakumar 2013). Resistance exercise training significantly improves strength and reduces depressive symptoms (Gordon et al. 2018). Reviews of yoga practice support its role as a self-soothing technique that can help modulate your stress response to both anxiety and depression (Harvard Health Publishing 2018). Refer to the resource list at the end of this chapter for more research findings.

Time to Master

- One week to assess your current activities, look for opportunities to exercise, and acknowledge your reasons for not exercising

- Eight weeks to gradually build up your exercise program

- Twelve weeks to establish the habit of doing a well-balanced exercise program

Instructions

Before reading further, complete the Exercise Inventory. Your answers will help you think about how you will create an exercise program tailored to your abilities, circumstances, and interests.

Exercise Inventory

1. How physically fit are you now? Circle the number that most applies to you on a scale of 1 to 10 (1 means "I'm really out of shape," 5 means "I exercise occasionally," and 10 means "I'm fit as a fiddle").

   1   2   3   4   5   6   7   8   9   10

2. How much time are you willing to spend exercising?

   Each day? _____

   Each week? _____

3. What time of day do you prefer to exercise? _____

4. How far are you willing to travel to exercise? _____
   _____

5. How much money are you willing or able to spend to exercise?

   How much on exercise equipment? _____

   How much on classes? _____

   How much on a club membership? _____

6. What exercise/activities have you tried in the past? _____
   _____

7. Which activities did you most enjoy? _____
   _____

8. Which activities did you least enjoy? _____
   _____

9. What motivates you to exercise? _____
   _____

10. Do you need a competitive edge (such as a competitive sport)? _____

   Do you prefer to exercise in a group (such as a class or a hiking group), with a friend (such as at the gym or while walking), or just by yourself (such as with in-home gym or equipment)? _____
   _____

11. Do you prefer indoor or outdoor activities? _____

12. How will you fit exercise into your current schedule? _____
   _____

13. Will you need to make changes in your routine during the week and/or on the weekends to add regular exercise? _____
   _____

Take Advantage of Opportunities to Exercise

Hopefully, by now, you appreciate the numerous benefits of exercise. You know you need to exercise more but don't seem to have enough time, opportunity, or motivation. Perhaps the biggest barrier to exercise is all the reasons going through your head—from boredom to being too tired to being too out of shape, the reasons you give yourself for not exercising are powerful. They are so powerful that they've succeeded in preventing you from meeting one of your basic needs. Use the next exercise to further assess your activity pattern and to confront what is preventing you from exercising.

Facing up to your excuses is an essential step to overcoming an inactive lifestyle. Keeping a daily Diary of Opportunities to Exercise will help you discover the times in your schedule when you can exercise regularly.

Here is a sample diary:

Angela's Diary of Opportunities to Exercise

Time	Opportunity to Exercise	Reasons for and Against Exercising
7:45 a.m.	Let dog out to run in the yard.	I could walk the dog but am running late.
8:15 a.m.	Drive to work.	I could bike to work, but it's too far and I can't because my bike has a flat.
10:00 a.m.	Drive with coworker to a special conference three blocks away.	I would have walked, but I couldn't very well say no to a friend offering a ride.
12:00 p.m.	Drive to lunch.	I want to save time. Besides, it looks like rain.
1:00 p.m.	Make calls to people who work on different floors of my building.	It's more efficient to phone.
3:00 p.m.	Walk to post office.	I need to stretch my legs.
5:00 p.m.	Collapse on sofa at home.	I could go jogging, but I'm exhausted and too out of shape since gaining those five pounds at Christmas.
7:30 p.m.	Back on the sofa.	I could walk the dog, but it's dark and this isn't a safe neighborhood. Also, I have a headache. Maybe tomorrow…

Visit http://www.newharbinger.com/43348 to download the Diary of Opportunities to Exercise and print three copies to fill out over the next few days. Make a note in your diary each time you have at least ten minutes free to take a walk or do some other kind of exercise. Note when you do exercise, and give reasons for exercising. Also, write down the things you say to yourself that hold you back or give you an excuse for not exercising.

Diary of Opportunities to Exercise

Time	Opportunity to Exercise	Reasons for and Against Exercising

When Angela reviewed her Diary of Opportunities to Exercise, she took a very close look at the reasons she was choosing not to exercise. Because she knew that these reasons were a barrier to doing something that she needed and wanted to do, she took the time to write out ways of overcoming these obstacles.

Angela's Responses to Reasons for Not Exercising

Reason for Not Exercising	Response or Solution
Running late…can't walk the dog.	*I rarely have time to walk the dog in the morning because I don't get up early enough to do it. I'll set the alarm fifteen minutes earlier and get up as soon as it goes off.*
Can't bike to work…flat tire.	*It's not a matter of "can't." I just don't want to bike to work. But I can fix the flat so that I can bike on weekends, when I do enjoy biking in the country.*
Couldn't decline a ride from a friend.	*This isn't true. Obviously I can say no, but sometimes I choose not to. I'll ask my friend to walk with me to meetings in the future.*
Save time by driving to lunch.	*An hour is plenty of time to walk to lunch, eat, and walk back.*
Drive to lunch because it looks like rain.	*This is the dumbest excuse yet! So what if it's cloudy? If I'm so concerned about the weather, I'll carry an umbrella or eat in the cafeteria downstairs.*
It's more efficient to phone.	*True, but face-to-face contact is valuable. And I do have the time to make the rounds in person.*
I'm too exhausted, out of shape, and overweight to jog.	*These are all signs of exercise deprivation and the very reasons why I should go jogging.*
The neighborhood is unsafe after dark.	*I could ask my husband to walk with me or do some indoor exercises or join a health club or plan my exercises for earlier in the day.*
I have a headache.	*Another possible sign of exercise deprivation and stress accumulation.*
Maybe tomorrow…	*My favorite strategy for avoiding exercise! I'll go walk the dog right now!*

Your Responses to Reasons for Not Exercising

Following Angela's example, write responses for your reasons not to exercise. For every reason you give not to exercise, think of how you might solve this problem.

Reason for Not Exercising	Response or Solution

Types of Exercise

There are four general categories of exercise:

- Endurance or aerobic: activities that increase your breathing and heart rate

- Strength and toning: exercises that build strong muscles and bones

- Balance: exercises that help prevent falls and avoid the disability that may result from falling

- Stretching and flexibility: exercises that give you more freedom of movement

Let's explore each type of exercise in depth along with some general recommendations for doing them.

Endurance or Aerobic Exercises

Aerobic exercises are repetitive and rhythmic. They involve sustained use of the large muscles in the body, especially in the legs and arms. The goals of aerobic exercise are to strengthen your cardiovascular system and to increase overall stamina. Aerobic exercise can improve the composition of the body by developing more lean body mass when working at your target heart rate. (Note: Instructions for determining your target heart rate are provided later in this chapter.) Endurance or aerobic exercises make you healthier overall.

Popular aerobic exercises include running, jogging, brisk walking, swimming, bicycling, and dancing. This wide array of choices offers alternatives to suit every lifestyle and range of physical conditions. You can measure the amount of exercise you are getting each day, including the number of steps in your normal daily activities, such as walking, climbing stairs, housecleaning, shopping, gardening, and mowing the lawn, by using a pedometer, a fitness tracker, or a phone app with a fitness tracker.

If you walk less than two miles per day (approximately two thousand steps are equivalent to one mile), consider yourself an inactive person and begin your exercise program slowly. The NIH reports that "adding a small and comfortable amount of walking, such as five to fifteen minutes two to three times per week, to one's usual daily activities has a low risk of musculoskeletal injury and no known risk of sudden severe cardiac events" (Physical Activity Guidelines Advisory Committee 2018, C-26). Adding bouts of physical activity of any length is also good for your health.

To create an endurance or aerobic exercise program, you need to consider frequency, duration, and intensity. *Frequency* is the number of sessions of moderate-to-vigorous exercise per day or per week, and *duration* is the amount of time spent per session. *Intensity* is the rate of energy expended per session, usually measured in MET-minutes (estimated metabolic equivalents of task), heart rate (beats per minute), or perceived rate of exertion. The NIH Physical Activity Guidelines Advisory

Committee (2018) recommends thirty to sixty minutes of moderately intense physical activity five out of seven days per week. It's better to increase frequency and duration before increasing intensity. The Mayo Clinic (2018) recommends getting "at least 150 minutes a week of moderate aerobic activity—such as brisk walking, swimming or mowing the lawn—or 75 minutes a week of vigorous aerobic activity—such as running or aerobic dancing."

Strength and Toning Exercises

Strength training involves maintaining or improving overall strength, endurance, and power in both muscles and bones. It's all about overcoming resistance, usually provided by free weights or machines, although some daily activities such as shoveling snow, climbing stairs, and lifting children or pets provide strength benefits as well. You want to consider the amount of resistance (strength), number of repetitions (endurance), and speed of movement (power) when setting goals and designing a program. Impact activities, such as running, jumping, and dancing, target bone health more directly. Toning exercises utilize higher repetitions and lower weights to target muscles that need firming. Examples are crunches for abdominal muscles, squats for thigh muscles, heel raises for calf muscles, and push-ups for arm and chest muscles. Muscle strengthening and increased bulk occur when larger weights and fewer repetitions are used.

There are three ways to strengthen and tone muscles: concentrically, isometrically, and eccentrically.

Concentrics involve the shortening of muscles against resistance through a range of movement. For example, your biceps concentrically shorten when you bend your elbow. Free weights, resistance bands, and the use of resistive weight machines are the most popular forms of concentric exercise. Concentric strengthening can be used to increase the size of the muscle or simply to tone it. Bigger muscles can provide more power, endurance, and speed. Toned muscles yield a firmer-looking body and are important for protecting joints. Concentric strengthening is a good way to gain and maintain the lean body mass that helps your body withstand the stresses of daily life.

Isometrics involve the contraction of muscles against resistance without any change in the length of the muscle fibers. For example, you can push your two hands together at chest level and feel your chest muscles tighten. Isometrics do not make muscles larger, but they do increase muscle strength.

Eccentrics involve the lengthening of muscles against resistance through a range of movement. For example, walking downstairs requires eccentric lengthening of the quadriceps (front thigh) muscles, whereas these same muscles must be concentrically shortened to walk upstairs.

There is general agreement in the evidence that progressive muscle strengthening exercises need to be done two to three nonconsecutive days per week and target all major muscle groups (legs, hips, back, abdomen, chest, shoulders, and arms) to be effective. Generally, one set of eight to twelve repetitions, performed to fatigue against challenging resistance, is effective for increasing muscular strength (Physical Activity Guidelines Advisory Committee 2018).

Balance Exercises

Balance exercises consist of positions, movements, and surfaces that test the body's postural system against gravity. Doing exercises seated is easier than standing, which is easier than walking. You can make balance exercises even more challenging when you close your eyes or move your arms in closer to your body and actually cross your arms over your chest. Likewise, bringing your feet closer together, standing with one foot in front of the other, or standing on one foot increases the challenge for your balance center and postural system. Finally, when you stand on a compliant surface, such as carpet, foam, or grass, instead of on a firm surface, your body will naturally sway in response to minute weight shifts through your feet on the surface. All of these positions, movements, and surface changes test and improve your balance. Having a strong core and strong leg muscles will further support and improve your overall balance.

Stretching and Flexibility Exercises

Stretching and flexibility exercises are used to increase muscle and joint flexibility. They are a good way to begin an exercise program and the easiest way to be mindful of stress and anxiety. Stretching exercises are also excellent for those who lead a sedentary life or are in poor physical condition. They help reawaken the body and prepare it to begin testing the benefits of aerobic, strengthening, and balance exercises.

Flexibility exercises need to be slow and sustained to enable muscles as well as tendons and ligaments in the joints to relax and stretch safely. They are most effective when held steady, without bouncing, for at least thirty seconds. Rhythmic breathing can help you observe the body relaxing. Stretching decreases muscle tension, improves circulation, and helps prevent injury during warm-ups and cooldowns before and after aerobic, strengthening, or balance exercises. Stretching is good to do whenever your body feels stressed, tense, stiff, or tired. And stretching before going to bed help relax and prepare the body for a good night's sleep

Setting Goals and Developing a Successful Program

A well-balanced exercise program includes each of the four exercise types discussed in the previous section. The President's Council on Sports, Fitness, and Nutrition (2017) recommends thirty minutes a day of physical activity for adults and sixty minutes a day for children, five days a week or more. If this seems overwhelming, try the following:

Phase 1: Begin doing something every day to increase your physical activity as part of your daily routine. Refer to your Diary of Opportunities to Exercise for some good examples of what you can do. It could be as simple as parking farther away from the entrance to your workplace or grocery store. Try this for a week. Be reassured that "it never hurts to start taking a little extra care when it comes to exercise…and general, overall wellness. And it doesn't take much" (Northwestern Medicine 2018). "About five minutes of aerobic exercise can begin to stimulate anti-anxiety effects" (Anxiety and Depression Association of America 2018).

Phase 2: Start walking five to fifteen minutes two to three times per week to build your endurance. Try this for three weeks.

Phase 3: Add some simple stretching, toning, and balance activities thirty or more minutes most days of the week. Add these activities for three more weeks and continue your walking program started in phase 2.

Phase 4: Decide whether you want to continue your walking program or if you want to add or substitute another aerobic activity, such as bicycling or swimming. Now is also the time to consider if you'd like to take up an amateur sport. Build up to at least thirty minutes of aerobic activity that makes you breathe hard on most days of the week.

Phase 5: Set up your weekly schedule with at least three exercise sessions per week that are comprised of exercises that are more or less consistent with what you want. Commit to sticking to this schedule over the next eight weeks.

If the idea of doing these five phases on your own still seems daunting, you may find it easier if you tell someone about your plan and ask that person to be your exercise buddy or to hold you accountable. If you have the resources, you can also consult with a personal trainer, preferably one who has an EIM credential (see Other Resources).

If your intention is to help manage your stress and anxiety over the long term, then it is time to set some goals and develop a plan to increase the amount of exercise you get during the day. Setting goals and writing them down will help you get started. First, review your answers to the questions in your Exercise Inventory, and think about the types of exercises you'd like to start with. Next, set SMART goals, which are detailed in the next section.

SMART Goals

SMART goals are specific, measurable, attainable, relevant, and time based. Be sure to consider your overall health, your current level of fitness, your age, the resources available to you, your time limitations, your personal interests, and your doctor's advice. Write your goals down and post them in a place where you'll see them every day. You will achieve success if you are consistent with your schedule, allowing for the fact that things will come up and you will need to adjust. Perfection is not the goal; be realistic. To ensure a successful start, it may help to set just one short-term goal for each week. Let's look at a couple of examples.

Example 1: Beginner. Bob wants to get back into exercise after a number of years without any regular program. He works hard at his day job and feels the stress of meeting the demands of a changing work environment. At the end of his workday, he feels too tired to exercise. He also feels the anxiety of providing for his growing family, and on weekends he wants to relax and spend time with them. He can't seem to find the time to get started with an exercise program. Here's Bob's plan to ease back into a regular exercise program; to make his workout more interesting, he decided to include a parcourse, which is an outdoor exercise course equipped with a series of stations to stop and perform a specific exercise along the way.

Exercise Goal	Frequency (times/week)	Duration (minutes/session)	Intensity (mild, moderate, vigorous)
1. *Park at the far edge of the lot at work*	*5 days this week*	*5-minute walk to work*	*Walk at mild-moderate pace*
2. *Continue goal #1 & walk during lunch*	*3 days/week for 3 weeks*	*10+ min/session*	*Walk at moderate pace*
3. *Continue goals #1 & #2; include parcourse*	*4 to 5 days/week for 3 weeks*	*30+ min/session*	*Walk at moderate-vigorous pace; parcourse mild-moderate pace*

Example 2: Reasonably fit. Sheila has been attending Zumba classes two times per week at her local gym and has taken thirty-minute walks most workdays at lunch for several years. Her doctor gives her two thumbs-up for both her exercise program and her low-normal blood pressure. However, since her fiftieth birthday, she has been dismayed by the effects of gravity on her physique. And she has been advised that she is at risk for developing osteoporosis, which only adds to the stress and anxiety she experiences in her already busy life. Thus, she would like to add a strengthening, stretching, and balance regimen but feels too overwhelmed to do the research and design it herself. She has decided that it is time to pay for the expertise of the physical therapist/personal trainer (PT) who consults at her gym. Here's Sheila's plan to take her exercise program to the next level.

Exercise Goal	Frequency (times/week)	Duration (minutes/session)	Intensity (mild, moderate, vigorous)
1. *Work with PT to develop full body program with free weights*	*3 times/week for 3 weeks*	*60 min/session*	*Moderate*

| 2. Continue PT program and substitute Zumba with tai chi | PT 3 days/ week; tai chi 2 days/week ongoing | 60 min/session | Moderate+ |
| 3. Continue goal #2 and add salsa dance class | Salsa 1 or 2 evenings/ week ongoing | Salsa classes are 60 min/ session with free dance an additional hour | Moderate-vigorous |

Setting SMART Goals

Write down three activity-exercise goals for the upcoming eight weeks. Refer back to phases 1 through 5 at the beginning of this section to get some ideas.

Exercise Goal	Frequency (times/week)	Duration (minutes/session)	Intensity (mild, moderate, vigorous)

Barriers are only as powerful as you allow them to be. If you can name your barriers and accept them as excuses, then you can tame them. Awareness is the first essential step in overcoming an inactive lifestyle. If you need help with improving and making your current exercise program more specifically appropriate and challenging, don't be afraid to ask for help. Consider taking a class or making an appointment with a personal trainer at a local gym or community center, or research your questions online or at your local library. If managing stress and anxiety are important priorities for you, then you will find ways to overcome your barriers and make the time to exercise.

Become curious and observant about your daily routine and take time to notice any opportunities to exercise. For example, while waiting for your carpool or public transportation, take those few moments to march in place, circle your shoulders, or try balancing on one leg. And don't be afraid to be silly and have fun while you're doing them. Invite others who are waiting to join you.

A few helpful hints as you seek success with your exercise program:

- Walking may be the best way to start if you are middle-aged, somewhat overweight, or have been relatively inactive.

- Swimming is good for people who are substantially overweight or have bone or joint problems.

- If you work with people all day, you may prefer exercise that you can do alone, such as walking, bicycling, or swimming.

- If you spend most of your day in solitary preoccupation with your work, you might prefer to make dates with friends to exercise or join a class.

- If tension is a normal part of your daily routine, you may benefit from an exercise that will help you let off steam, such as kickboxing or a martial art, or a competitive sport like basketball or tennis.

- If you feel empty or low by the end of your workday, then centering exercises like yoga, qi gong, or tai chi may be just what you need.

If a negative view of yourself is holding you back and keeping you trapped in a sedentary lifestyle, know that you are not alone. Such beliefs make it hard for any of us to initiate an exercise program on our own. One way to counter a negative self-image is to get together with a trusted friend who already exercises regularly. This friend can be your ally, your cheerleader, who encourages you to get started and to stick with a program. Another option is to join an exercise group or class that will provide ongoing support, instruction, and a predictable routine. Remember that exercise is important and available for all ages, sizes, and shapes.

If you are afraid of injuring yourself, then first get cleared by your primary care provider. An experienced professional can also help you design a safe and effective exercise program. Likewise, many books and classes can provide information about how to exercise safely, what to expect as you progress, and how to cope with any difficulties you encounter along the way. There is also a list of useful resources at the end of this chapter.

Special Considerations

As you set about preparing to implement your exercise program, here are some practical tips:

- Time of day offers different advantages and disadvantages in terms of temperatures and distractions.

- When exercising outdoors on cold days, be sure to wear several layers of clothing, mittens or gloves, and a hat to prevent heat loss.

- Cold rainy weather can increase your risk of hypothermia. Be alert to the symptoms, which include intense shivering, lack of coordination, slurred speech, and extreme fatigue.

- Drink more water when you exercise in the sun. Staying hydrated is essential. Symptoms of dehydration include lack of sweat, shriveled and dry skin, muscle cramps, dry eyes or blurred vision, headache or feelings of confusion or disorientation, and extreme fatigue.

- On hot, humid days, you should sweat a lot, and you need to drink lots of water. If sweating stops, your body temperature can become dangerously high.

- Be familiar with the symptoms of heatstroke, which include feelings of dizziness or light-headedness, weakness or muscle cramps, a throbbing headache, red/hot/dry skin, a rapid heartbeat, and rapid shallow breathing.

- If you must exercise at night on city streets, be sure to wear reflective clothing, travel on well-lit streets, and carry identification, a loud whistle, and a cell phone. This is an excellent time to exercise with a friend.

- Plan to exercise before meals or at least two hours after your last meal.

- Tell your friends, family, and coworkers about your exercise plan, so they can provide support and encouragement to help you stay on track.

- Variety is the spice of life, so be sure to choose more than one type of exercise activity, even something fun, to minimize the possibility of boredom.

Warm Up and Prepare Your Body for Exercise

Always start with gentle warm-up stretches to avoid putting unnecessary stress on your body and joints. Warm-up exercises increase your metabolism and your body temperature. The increase in blood flow and oxygen to your muscles, heart, and lungs helps prepare your body for more vigorous exercise. Warm-ups also decrease your chance of injury or cramping and can lessen overall muscle soreness. Start with ten minutes of stretching before you begin your workout. If your body likes it and wants it (and you have the time for it), do more. Gentle reminder: hold each stretch for thirty seconds.

Do Aerobic Exercise Within Your Target Heart Rate Zone

As you do your aerobic workout, your large skeletal muscles rhythmically tense and relax, stimulating the blood flow through your arteries, veins, heart, and lungs. Your heart rate is particularly important. Much like the speedometer in your car helps you monitor how fast you are going, your heart rate tells you how hard you are working and whether you should work harder or not during aerobic exercise.

A normal resting pulse may range from forty to one hundred beats per minute, depending on your level of physical fitness. To benefit from aerobic exercise, your heart must reach and stay within a range known as your *target heart rate zone* for at least twenty minutes: this is the safest exercise range for your heart while you are exercising. At this pace, the relaxation response is stimulated, which helps manage stress and anxiety.

Many exercise machines have a heart rate monitor, which shows your heart rate as you exercise. You can also find out how fast your heart is working by simply taking your pulse. If you are unfamiliar with monitoring your heart rate, start practicing by taking your pulse while sitting quietly. Turn the palm of your right hand toward your body. Place the fingertips of your left index and middle fingers firmly on your right wrist near the bone that joins your thumb to your wrist. You will feel your pulse. To determine your heart rate for one minute, take your pulse for ten seconds and multiply the number by six.

The American Heart Association (2018) recommends doing aerobic exercise within your target heart rate zone. Calculate your maximum heart rate by subtracting your age from 220. Then multiply your maximum heart rate by 50 percent and by 85 percent to find your target heart rate zone. Exercising within this range provides a safe way to progress, placing moderate stress on your heart. This stress is considered a positive stress and one that strengthens your heart muscle to improve its efficiency. By monitoring your heart rate during exercise and comparing it to your target rate, you'll have immediate feedback about whether you are doing too much or too little exercise. If your heart rate is greater than your target rate, you slow down; if your heart rate is lower than your target rate, you speed up.

Cool Down After Aerobics

Allow your body to return safely to its normal state after you finish exercising. A period of cooling down helps decrease your metabolism and body temperature and slows down your heart rate. Likewise, a cooldown helps prevent muscle soreness. When jogging or running, always end your session with five minutes of slow walking. Take long exaggerated steps, stretching your legs. Let your arms dangle loosely, and shake your hands. The stretching and toning exercises that you used as warm-ups can be used for cooling down as well. Spend about ten minutes doing stretches after your workout.

Avoiding Injury

Here are a few suggestions to decrease your chances of injury:

- Have a physical checkup. Get cleared by your doctor or primary health care provider before beginning a regular exercise program. This is especially important if you are older, out of shape, obese, recovering from a serious illness or operation, or are taking medications that require regular checkups.

- Follow any special precautions suggested by your doctor or health care provider.

- Start slowly and build up gradually. Progress at a steady pace.

- Set realistic goals and monitor your progress.

- Spread your exercise over the week rather than becoming a weekend warrior who only exercises on weekends.

- Exercise within your target heart rate zone. A general rule of thumb is to walk and talk while exercising at a moderate rate. Always warm up before moderate to vigorous exercises and cool down afterward.

- Drink plenty of fluids to replace any fluids lost during vigorous exercise.

- Don't exercise if you are feeling sick. Your body needs rest to recover.

- Don't exercise after a large meal, because blood flow to the large muscles is limited.

- Don't use ankle or arm weights if you have low back pain or knee or ankle problems. Weights place added stress on your back and joints.

- Wear comfortable shoes that offer good support to your feet and ankles. It is generally recommended that you replace your running shoes every four hundred to six hundred miles or every six months.

- Wear comfortable, lightweight, loose-fitting layers of clothing. Be prepared to remove clothing as your body temperature increases during the warm-up and aerobic phases and to add clothing as your body temperature decreases when you are cooling down.

- Listen to your body. Although you may experience some soreness after the first few times you exercise, you should not experience acute or sharp pain.

Contact your doctor or primary health care provider once you have begun your exercise program if you develop any of the following symptoms:

- Your heart rate becomes irregular and begins to skip beats.

- Your heart rate takes longer than fifteen minutes to slow down to its normal resting rate.

- You feel a tightness, pressure, or pain in your chest, shoulders, arms, or neck.

- You feel dizzy or nauseated.

- You feel extreme breathlessness after only mild exertion.

- You feel exhausted long after your exercise session is over.

- You experience acute or sharp pain anywhere in your body whenever you exercise.

Sticking with It

There are two major obstacles to overcome when starting an exercise program. The first is to just get started. The second is to keep at it. If you have followed the instructions in the preceding sections, you've jumped the first hurdle. The second may be more difficult. Choose exercise activities that you enjoy doing and cross-train so that you have more than one activity from which to choose. Visualize success and stay with your exercise program until it becomes a routine part of your day.

You may find the following Exercise Diary helpful. Fill it out every day for several weeks, and you will be well on your way to recognizing the benefits of including exercise as a regular part of your life. Each day that you exercise, fill in the activity, location, distance or duration, and any comments, thoughts, or feelings you have after completing the exercise. Visit http://www.newharbinger.com/43348 to download this Exercise Diary form.

Exercise Diary

Week of _____

Target heart rate: _____

Friendly reminder: Warm up and cool down.

Day	Activity	Location	Distance or Duration	Comments, Thoughts, Feelings
Monday				
Tuesday				
Wednesday				
Thursday				
Friday				
Saturday				
Sunday				

Congratulations! You are busy. And you are choosing to exercise! Exercise is an especially important outlet to relieve the pressures of daily life. Without exercise, our ability to cope with everyday stress is jeopardized. Exercise not only keeps our bodies fit, flexible, and strong but also gives us energy, keeps our minds alert, and gives us the balance and resilience needed to make us capable of handling any stress that comes along.

Further Reading

American College of Sports Medicine. 2014. "Exercise Is Medicine Fact Sheet." http://exerciseismedicine .org/assets/page_documents/EIMFactSheet_2014.pdf.

American Heart Association. 2018. "Know Your Target Heart Rates for Exercise, Losing Weight, and Health." http://www.heart.org/en/healthy-living/fitness/fitness-basics/target-heart-rates.

Anderson E., and G. Shivakumar. 2013. "Effects of Exercise and Physical Activity on Anxiety." *Frontiers in Psychiatry* 4: 27.

Anxiety and Depression Association of America. 2018. "Exercise for Stress and Anxiety." https://adaa.org /living-with-anxiety/managing-anxiety/exercise-stress-and-anxiety#.

Gordon, B. R., C. P. McDowell, M. Hallgren, J. D. Meyer, M. Lyons, and M. P. Herring. 2018. "Association of Efficacy of Resistance Exercise Training with Depressive Symptoms: Meta-Analysis and Meta-Regression Analysis of Randomized Clinical Trials." *JAMA Psychiatry* 75 (6): 566–76.

Harvard Health Publishing. 2018. "Yoga for Anxiety and Depression." Published April 2009. Updated May 9. *Harvard Mental Health Letter.* https://www.health.harvard.edu/mind-and-mood/yoga-for-anxiety -and-depression.

Johns Hopkins Medicine. 2018. "Stressed Out? Five Ways for Women to Stay Heart Healthy." https://www .hopkinsmedicine.org/health/healthy-woman/mind-mood/stressed-out-5-tips-for-women-to -stay-heart-healthy.

Laskowski, E. R. 2018. "What Are the Risks of Sitting Too Much?" Mayo Clinic Healthy Lifestyle, Adult Health. https://www.mayoclinic.org/healthy-lifestyle/adult-health/expert-answers/sitting/faq-20058005.

Mayo Clinic. 2018. "Exercise Intensity: How to Measure It." https://www.mayoclinic.org/healthy-lifestyle/ fitness/in-depth/exercise-intensity/art-20046887.

Northwestern Medicine. 2018. "Four Ways to Alleviate Anxiety." http://www.nmbreakthroughs.org/ emotional-health/4-ways-to-reduce-anxiety.

Physical Activity Guidelines Advisory Committee. 2018. "2018 Physical Activity Guidelines Advisory Committee Scientific Report." Washington, DC: US Department of Health and Human Services.

President's Council on Sports, Fitness, and Nutrition. 2017. "Ways to Be Active." US Department of Health and Human Services. https://www.hhs.gov/fitness/be-active/ways-to-be-active/index.html.

Teychenne, M., S. A. Costigan, and K. Parker. 2015. "The Association Between Sedentary Behaviour and Risk of Anxiety: A Systematic Review." *BMC Public Health* 15: 513.

Other Resources

Many groups have information about physical activity and exercise. The following list of resources will help you get started:

AMERICAN COLLEGE OF SPORTS MEDICINE
    Phone: 317–637–9200
    http://www.acsm.org

AMERICAN COUNCIL ON EXERCISE
    Phone: 888–825–3636
    http://www.acefitness.org

CENTERS FOR DISEASE CONTROL AND PREVENTION
    Phone: 800–232–4636
    TTY: 888–232–6348
    http://www.cdc.gov

CLEVELAND CLINIC STRESS MEDITATIONS
    Offers a meditation app with relaxation techniques.
    https://my.clevelandclinic.org/mobile-apps/stress-free-now-app

EXERCISE IS MEDICINE
    Lists qualified exercise professionals with the EIM (Exercise Is Medicine) credential.
    http://www.exerciseismedicine.org

KAISER PERMANENTE THRIVE
    Online Health Encyclopedia for over four thousand health topics.
    http://kp.org/stressmanagement

MAYO CLINIC
    Website offers tips on stress management and relief.
    https://www.mayoclinic.org/healthy-lifestyle/stress-management/basics/stress-relief
    /hlv-20049495

MEDLINEPLUS
    National Library of Medicine
    http://www.medlineplus.gov

NATIONAL COUNCIL ON AGING
    Phone: 571–527–3900
    http://www.benefitscheckup.org

NATIONAL INSTITUTE ON AGING

Go4Life offers free, evidence-based resources for older adults in one convenient place.
https://www.nia.nih.gov/health/exercise-physical-activity

PRESIDENT'S COUNCIL ON SPORTS, FITNESS, AND NUTRITION

Phone: 240–276–9567
http://www.fitness.gov

CHAPTER 21

When It Doesn't Come Easy—Getting Unstuck

This book has covered many techniques to reduce stress and tension. Essentially, they provide alternatives to your old stressful habits. You may have found that just practicing the new skills and observing the positive effects has caused you to give up your old habits. For instance, you may have found that practicing slow, deep breaths rather than short, constricted breaths results in a relaxed sense of well-being. This positive feedback from your body may have provided ample motivation for you to give up your old anxiety-provoking shallow breathing habit. However, if you are like most people, at some point you probably encountered some difficulty in exchanging familiar old habits for new ones. This chapter takes a look at why old habits are hard to part with, even when they are obviously contributing to your stress. It also offers some suggestions for how to deal with your own resistance to change.

If you find yourself skipping an exercise session you have contracted with yourself to do, or you are aware that you are just going through the motions of the exercises, it is time for an intervention with yourself. Ask yourself the following questions:

1. Why am I doing these exercises? What outcome do I want?

2. Are these reasons really important to me?

3. What am I doing or would I like to be doing instead of these exercises?

4. Is this alternative activity more important to me than doing the exercises is?

5. Can I schedule my life so that I can do the exercises *and* this alternative activity?

6. If I do not want to do the exercises now, exactly when and where will I do them next?

7. What would I have to give up if I succeeded with my exercises?

8. What or whom would I have to confront if I succeeded with my exercises?

Chapter 16, "Goal Setting and Time Management," covers many topics that could help you get back on track by (1) clarifying what is most important to you, (2) setting goals, (3) developing an action plan, (4) evaluating how you spend your time, (5) combating procrastination, (6) organizing and prioritizing your time, and (7) dealing with overstimulation.

Taking Responsibility for Your Decisions

It is difficult to learn new habits on your own when, at first, the rewards for your efforts may be minimal. When distractions occur, decide whether you want to be detoured or to continue on your chosen route. If you decide to take the detour, do so with full awareness after weighing the pros and cons. Before going off on the detour, make an appointment with yourself for when and where you are next going to do your exercises. In this way, you take responsibility for your decision. In addition, you are less likely to feel bad about yourself for not following through on your original plan, if that is your conscious choice.

What are the reasons you give yourself for skipping your exercises? Typical reasons are "I'm too busy today," "I'm too tired," "Missing once won't hurt," "Another person needs my help," "This isn't working," "This is boring," "I feel relaxed and unstressed today, so I don't need to exercise," or "I feel too bad today to do the exercises." These excuses are seductive because they are partially true. That is, you may really feel very busy or tired, somebody may need your help, and missing one session probably won't hurt. The part that isn't true is the implication that because you are busy or tired or someone needs your help, you cannot do the exercise sessions. A more truthful statement would be "I am tired. I could do the exercises, but I choose not to," or "I could do my exercises, but I choose to help my friend rather than do them." The important point here is that you take responsibility for your decision to choose one activity over another rather than pretend that you are the passive victim of circumstances such as your fatigue, your friend's demands, or any other priorities that keep you busy. You are in charge of your own life balance.

Confront Your Excuses

The excuses you give yourself for not doing your exercises are likely to be the same ones that you've used for years to keep yourself locked into a stressful situation. These excuses are based on faulty premises. For example, a busy executive firmly believed she had no right to relax until all her work was done. She thought that if she ever took some time for herself, her department would not achieve the goals and outcomes she had agreed to meet each year. Over the years, she became anxious and depressed, had difficulty maintaining relationships, and developed a number of physical complaints. Her perfectionist belief that she personally had to oversee all of the work in her department before she could ever have time to relax had caused a gradual depletion of her energy. Realistically, the work is never done; therefore, she could never relax.

But she had overlooked her innate right (some would call it an obligation) to relax and replenish her vital store of energy. This woman had defined her priorities as being "executive first and me second," without taking into account the importance of maintaining good mental and physical health by relaxing and getting away from stressful activities for a while. If you, like this woman, say to yourself, *I'm indispensable. Important things won't get done without me and may even fall apart*, consider putting your mental and physical health at the top of your list of priorities. The key to productivity and good health is to create balance in your life.

If you are an energetic person who likes to get things done yesterday, when working with these exercises, slow down your pace. Having to prove yourself or needing to rush can only create stress. Enthusiasm may push you to take on too many exercises at once or to do the sessions for too long a time. When you do too much too fast, you run a high risk of burning out and losing interest. Furthermore, you are likely to feel guilty for not keeping up with the rigorous program you've set for yourself, once your early enthusiasm calms down. Soon you will find yourself coming up with excuses to avoid doing your exercises at all (*I'm overextended already in so many areas of my life. Why should I add to my burden?*). In addition, you may feel confused when you begin to experience having more energy as a result of doing the relaxation and stress reduction exercises. Resist the temptation to pour this extra energy back into your work. Rather, use it for further rest and enjoyment.

If you find yourself saying things like "I just don't feel like doing it today, maybe I will tomorrow..." day after day, give yourself a good mental kick or talking-to. It is simply not true that you must be motivated to do something before you do it. Motivation is often sparked by action. For example, if you take a brisk ten-minute walk, you are likely to feel good from the results and want to continue. Tell yourself that you have to do an activity for only five or ten minutes. Often, once you are into an activity, the momentum of doing it will carry you through to its completion.

At the very least, without feeling an ounce of motivation, you can work on a project for five or ten minutes a day until it is done. Sometimes, lack of motivation is a symptom of depression. However, depression often improves when you become more active. Tell yourself, *Of course I don't feel like doing it. So what? Do it anyway!*

Confronting Roadblocks to Stress Management and Relaxation

If you read this workbook without doing any of the exercises, it's likely that you are only dabbling. Intellectually, you see the value of the exercises, but, somehow, you never get much past the stage of thinking about them; or you may actually do some of the exercises but never apply them to everyday situations. For the dabbler, this is just another book with some interesting ideas rather than a workbook promoting new ways of experiential learning to deal with stress.

Some people are frightened by novel experiences, and their fear becomes a roadblock to their success. You might become overwhelmed by some side effect of a relaxation technique, such as tingling in your arms and legs. Unfortunately, you may then stop the exercise instead of going on to find that the tingling isn't harmful and that it disappears with time. You can get turned off by a single element of an exercise and, rather than changing the exercise to fit your needs, you may drop the entire exercise. Perhaps you don't understand a step in the instructions and, rather than ad-lib, you chuck the whole thing. It can be a valuable growth experience to work through these difficulties on your own or to find a friend who would be willing to interpret and do the exercises with you.

When Symptoms Persist

Sometimes stress symptoms persist in spite of regular relaxation and stress reduction work. If you are a conscientious person and have been practicing regularly, this can be disheartening. Here are a few reasons why this might be happening to you.

Are You Suggestible?

Some people are highly suggestible, and once they learn about symptoms, they begin to experience every one they hear about. For example, one very tense policeman joined a relaxation group to overcome his tendency to hyperventilate when under stress. He began to experience all of the physical symptoms described by the other group members: migraines, lower back pain, rapid heartbeat, and so forth. Doing deep breathing or using his coping skills training helped him combat these tendencies.

Do You Receive Some Benefit from Your Symptoms?

A surprising number of people are attached to their symptoms, which often serve a very definite purpose. For example, your headaches may get you out of interpersonal situations you want to avoid without having to take the responsibility of disappointing others. By keeping a log noting when your symptoms first appear and the activities (or would-be activities) that surround them, you can find out whether your symptoms rescue you from more unpleasant experiences. If you suspect that your symptoms provide you with a secondary gain in this manner, refer to chapter 17, "Assertiveness Training." It should provide you with the incentive and the tools to learn to be more direct in saying no, rather than having to resort to the discomfort of stress symptoms.

Are Your Symptoms a Reminder That You Need to Change Something?

Your symptoms of tension may be a signal that you are not dealing effectively with something in your life and that you are covering up your feelings. For example, you may be angry with your family but not sharing this fact with them. You might be putting off talking about a particular conflict because you don't see any way to improve matters. For example, a nurse was visited every other weekend by her very spoiled, demanding stepdaughter. The nurse had agreed to the arrangement when she married, and now she felt trapped by it. Over the course of three years, the visits from her stepdaughter invariably produced a migraine headache. To counteract this symptom, she finally negotiated a new deal with her husband, which allowed her to spend Sundays on her own, away from home, while he spent the day with his daughter.

The people around you may very well be aware that you are withholding stressful feelings and that something is wrong. Nevertheless, they cannot read your mind and are unlikely to come to your rescue. You know best what you need. Letting others know your feelings and what you want opens the way to engaging them in helping you make a change.

Can You Find Other Ways to Take Care of Yourself?

Your symptoms may be your way of getting others to take care of you when you feel you cannot directly ask for help or for extra consideration. If you are tired and have a bad backache, someone else will have to do the cooking and cleaning, while keeping the house quiet. Ask yourself when your symptoms first began. What was going on in your life that might have contributed to them? One retired woman who had suffered from periodic colitis since early childhood recalled that her abdominal cramping had begun when her younger twin brothers were born. She remembered that the only time her busy mother ever had to hold and rock her was when she was suffering from the early symptoms of colitis. As an adult, she noted that she tended to get colitis symptoms only when her husband was away and left her alone in the evenings.

Does Your Way of Dealing with Stress Remind You of Someone Else in Your Life?

It is possible that you've developed a stress symptom similar to that of an important person in your life as part of your identification with that person. For example, you may have learned not only to be hardworking and successful from your father but also to deal with stress in a manner similar to the way he does. For example, carrying your tension in your jaw, you may come to the point of grinding your teeth just like your father does. Since characteristic ways of responding to stress are generally learned, ask yourself who in your family shares your symptoms. It's often easier to see how your relatives are not dealing effectively with the stress in their lives than to see it in yourself. The next step is to observe and see if the same is true for you.

If you continue having difficulty reducing the stress in your life, consider consulting a professional. You may be interested in one-on-one psychotherapy sessions or in joining a relaxation and stress reduction group. Your doctor, company health plan, community health organization, local community college, and adult education programs are all good places to start looking for professional help.

Persistence Pays

Finally, don't give up. Your ability to relax, learn to handle stress, and heal yourself can be tremendously empowering. Change might not always come easy—you may feel stuck in your old stressful habits—but you can do it. All it takes is patience, persistence, a commitment to yourself...and time.

Martha Davis, PhD, was a psychologist in the department of psychiatry at Kaiser Permanente Medical Center in Santa Clara, CA, where she practiced individual, couples, and group psychotherapy for more than thirty years prior to her retirement. She is coauthor of *Thoughts and Feelings*.

Elizabeth Robbins Eshelman, MSW, worked for the Kaiser Permanente Health Care Program for thirty-seven years. During her tenure, she was a clinical social worker, hospice director, researcher, health educator, and management development instructor and coach. She is retired and lives in Northern California.

Matthew McKay, PhD, is a professor at the Wright Institute in Berkeley, CA. He has authored and coauthored numerous books, including *Self-Esteem*, *Thoughts and Feelings*, *When Anger Hurts*, and *ACT on Life Not on Anger*. McKay received his PhD in clinical psychology from the California School of Professional Psychology, and specializes in the cognitive behavioral treatment of anxiety and depression. He lives and works in the greater San Francisco Bay Area.

Index

MORE BOOKS *from*
NEW HARBINGER PUBLICATIONS

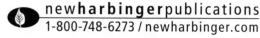

Register your **new harbinger** titles for additional benefits!

When you register your **new harbinger** title—purchased in any format, from any source—you get access to benefits like the following:

- Downloadable accessories like printable worksheets and extra content

- Instructional videos and audio files

- Information about updates, corrections, and new editions

Not every title has accessories, but we're adding new material all the time.

Access free accessories in 3 easy steps:

1. Sign in at NewHarbinger.com (or **register** to create an account).

2. Click on **register a book**. Search for your title and click the **register** button when it appears.

3. Click on the **book cover or title** to go to its details page. Click on **accessories** to view and access files.

That's all there is to it!

If you need help, visit:

NewHarbinger.com/accessories

new harbinger
CELEBRATING
40 YEARS